Emerging Trends in

Cartilage Tympanoplasty

Tragal cartilage with open perichondrium flap

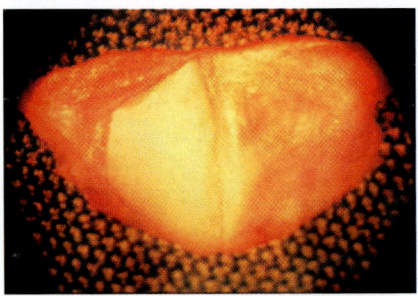

Emerging Trends in
Cartilage
Tympanoplasty

KK Desarda
MS (ORL), FACS (ORL), DLO (Lond)

Professor Emeritus and Head
Otolaryngology
BJ Medical College and
KEM Hospital, Pune

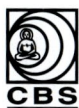

CBS Publishers & Distributors Pvt Ltd

New Delhi • Bengaluru • Chennai • Kochi • Kolkata • Mumbai
Hyderabad • Nagpur • Patna • Pune • Vijayawada

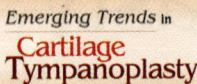

Emerging Trends in
Cartilage
Tympanoplasty

ISBN: 978-81-239-2948-4

Copyright © Author and Publisher

First Edition: **2016**

Published by Satish Kumar Jain and produced by Varun Jain for
CBS Publishers & Distributors Pvt Ltd
4819/XI Prahlad Street, 24 Ansari Road, Daryaganj, New Delhi 110 002, India.
Ph: 23289259, 23266861, 23266867   Fax: 011-23243014
Website: www.cbspd.com   e-mail: delhi@cbspd.com; cbspubs@airtelmail.in.
Corporate Office: 204 FIE, Industrial Area, Patparganj, Delhi 110 092
Ph: 4934 4934   Fax: 4934 4935   e-mail: publishing@cbspd.com;
                                               publicity@cbspd.com

Branches

- **Bengaluru:** Seema House 2975, 17th Cross, K.R. Road, Banasankari 2nd Stage, Bengaluru 560 070, Karnataka
  Ph: +91-80-26771678/79   Fax: +91-80-26771680   e-mail: bangalore@cbspd.com
- **Chennai:** 7, Subbaraya Street, Shenoy Nagar, Chennai 600 030, Tamil Nadu
  Ph: +91-44-26680620, 26681266   Fax: +91-44-42032115   e-mail: chennai@cbspd.com
- **Kochi:** Ashana House, 39/1904, AM Thomas Road, Valanjambalam, Eranakulam 682 018, Kochi, Kerala
  Ph: +91-484-4059061-62-64-65   Fax: +91-484-4059065   e-mail: kochi@cbspd.com
- **Kolkata:** No. 6/B, Ground Floor, Rameswar Shaw Road, Kolkata 700 014, West Bengal
  Ph: +91-33-2289-1126, 1127, 1128,   e-mail: Kolkata@cbspd.com
- **Mumbai:** 83-C, Dr E Moses Road, Worli, Mumbai-400018, Maharashtra
  Ph: +91-22-24902340/41   Fax: +91-22-24902342   e-mail: mumbai@cbspd.com

Representatives

• **Hyderabad**	0-9885175004	• **Nagpur**	0-9021734563	• **Patna**	0-9334159340
• **Pune**	0-9623451994	• **Vijayawada**	0-9000660880		

Printed at: Magic International, Greater Noida, UP

to
my wife **Sheela**
and
daughters, **Chetana** and Shilpa
who made it all worthwhile

Foreword

It is a pleasure and an honor for me to write the Foreword to this remarkable monograph on emerging trends in cartilage tympanoplasty as used by Prof KK Desarda during the last 30 years.

In 600 patients, Prof Desarda used four techniques — the inlay butterfly graft technique, the cartilage–perichondrium composite island graft technique, the palisade technique and the cartilage shield technique.

Besides the clear description of the cartilage–perichondrium tympanoplasty methods, the author in a clear way has described in detail the middle ear surgical anatomy, physiology of sound transformer mechanism, surgical pathology and pathogenesis of reperforations. The principles in reconstructive tympanoplasty and use of various graft materials have been described in detail.

The author has also described why cartilage perichondrium is an ideal graft in reconstructive tympanoplasty and the advantages of cartilage in ossiculoplasty and mastoid obliteration.

Prof Desarda has concluded the monograph with the fact that cartilage–perichondrium is an ideal and very useful graft for the reconstruction of middle ear pathology. Based on my experience in cartilage tympanoplasty, I fully agree with this conclusion, and even believe that cartilage tympanoplasty will become most common middle ear surgery, with many new methods. Therefore, we should honor the pioneers of cartilage tympanoplasty, like Prof Desarda.

Mirko Tos MD PhD
Chairman and Professor
Department of Otorhinolaryngology
Gentofte Hospital
University of Copenhagen
Denmark

Preface

The purpose of writing this monograph is to provide an assessment of the current state-of-art in reconstructive cartilage tympanoplasty using cartilage as a composite graft. For past fifty years, the invention of the operating microscope, refinements in anaesthesia, and the introduction of antibiotics have led to considerable improvements in the treatment of chronic middle ear diseases. Interest in devising better methods of management has stimulated the development of a new system of surgical treatment

In recent years cartilage tympanoplasties have been used more and more often in otosurgical practice and several new methods have been published. It has been my main interest to analyze the anatomical and functional results of surgery for illustrating functional differences between the various methods and to promote clinical and basic research in cartilage tympanoplasty.

The task of bringing out this monograph not only involves making alterations and additions but to have the most innovative and challenging newer techniques and newer metods in cartilage tympanoplasty for achieving the best results. The technical modifications in different pathological conditions and in difficult situations are well discussed in the surgical procedures with its solutions. The fate of the cartilage graft is discussed in detail with its histochemistry studied by electron mircroscpe by various otosurgeons.

This study includes 600 cases of varied middle ear pathologies, both safe and unsafe types, such as perforations, cholesteatoma, atelectatic, retraction pockets, ossicular deformities, and recurrent mastoid cavity problems. I have tried to explore the latest updates, newer techniques and methods of various composite grafts in the management of cartilage tympanoplasty and also discussed the satisfactory solutions

In this monograph I have included a very interesting chapter on efficacy of evicel (Fibrin-sealant) in composite graft tympanoplasty. This is a recent development in cartilage–perichondrium grafting. I have also included a chapter on the current concepts in paediatric cartilage tympanoplasty which I am sure otologists will accept in their clinical practice. The another inclusion is the colour atlas of otoscopy for easy understanding of the pathological conditions and making a decision in various methods in cartilage tympanoplasty.

With these few words I would like to present this monograph to our readers and hope it will stimulate the experienced otologists to a greater height.

KK Desarda

Acknowledgements

It is the wealth of experience and knowledge that is generated within the portals of the KEM Hospital Research Centre, Pune, and the commitment that this hospital has made towards the dissemination of knowledge through education, that has provided me with the opportunity to write this monograph.

The gratitude I feel towards this institution can hardly be put into words. It is with this profound sense of gratitude that I thank the management of KEM Hospital, the Medical Director, Academic Director, Research Director, Medical Administrator, nursing staff of OT and OPD, and very pertinently the patients without whom this monograph would not have been possible.

A special mention of Prof DM Anklesaria, consultant ENT surgeon, Mumbai, who is an excellent teacher, mentor and inspiring force in the preparation of this monograph. I deeply appreciate his advice throughout the preparation of the monograph.

Thanks are due to Prof Plester, Prof Hems, Prof Steinbach, Prof Hildmann and Prof Pusalkar for their innovative work in cartilage tympanoplasty which inspired me to take up this study which has now become the monograph for the faculty of otolaryngology.

I extend my sincere thanks to Prof Mirko Tos, Chairman and Professor, Department of Otorhinolaryngology, Gentofte Hospital, University of Copenhegan, Denmark, for appreciating the text and writing the Foreword to this monograph. I also appreciate his excellent drawings in various methods of cartilage tympanoplasties which helped me in the preparation of this monograph.

I deeply appreciate the review of literature given by JL Dornhoffer on cartilage tympanoplasty which helped me a lot in the preparation of this monograph. His diagrammatic illustrations were eye-catching for understanding the various techniques in cartilage tympanoplasty.

Special thanks must be made for the constant support and dedicated assistance of my postgraduate students who have contributed in collecting the material, cases, data analysis, and pre- and postoperative management of all patients subjected for this study.

I extend my sincere thanks to my department staff with whose inspiration I could complete this monograph.

Thanks are also due for Johnson & Johnson Co Pvt Ltd for providing Evicel product for clinical application in cartilage tympanoplasty which gave excellent results in graft take up in our study.

I appreciate the help given by Mrs Sadhana Lokare and Mr Rajesh from research centre in organizing the computer work during the preparation of this book. I cannot forget our Librarian, Miss Vaishali Kulkarni, for collecting the references and timely help despite her busy working.

Last but not least I extend sincere thanks to CBS Publishers & Distributors Pvt Ltd, New Delhi, for accepting this monograph for publication and for the cooperation in bringing out this monograph.

KK Desarda

Contents

Introduction

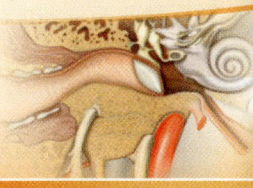

1

The first known attempt to repair an eardrum perforation was allegedly made by Banzer, in 1640, using a swine bladder membrane graft. In 1853, Toynbee introduced the "artificial eardrum", a small rubber disc with a silver rod—to facilitate introduction and extraction. In 1878, Berthold used a skin graft and in 1887, Blake recommended the use of a piece of paper as a template to tympanic membrane regeneration. Notwithstanding, it was only after 1944, with the beginning of antibiotics and with the improvement in surgical techniques that other materials were used as grafts in tympanoplasties. After this time, in 1952, Zollner and Wullstein published their methods, using retroauricular skin grafts; however, they did not succeed in treating tympanic membrane perforations.

Brazilian data, published by Costa in 1976, showed good results in the treatment of tympanic membrane perforations with the use of temporal fascia grafts and dura mater grafts. In 1983, Miniti showed a significant audiometric improvement in patients submitted to tympanic membrane repair surgery with the use of dura mater. In 2003, Oliveira observed that the use of synthetic biomaterial (latex biomembrane with polylysine) could contribute to a greater graft take rate of temporal fascia in tympanoplasties.

Thus, numerous types of tympanoplasty grafts have been described. The most commonly used techniques for graft placement on the tympanic membrane are the "underlay" (medial) and "onlay" (lateral), and the most used types of graft are the temporal muscle fascia and perichondrium, with similar success rates (approximately 90%).

A dry and instant hearing apparatus is an essential prerequisite for normal hearing. The earliest reconstructive surgeries were tried in the 16th and 18th centuries. However, tympanoplasty was introduced in a systematic form by Wullstein and Zollner in the early fifties, even then little attempt was made to reconstruct the middle ear sound transformer mechanism. An open cavity was the rules, as was a shallow middle ear space. Results were frequently unsatisfactory. With the development of tympanoplasty techniques, equal attention was given to the reconstruction of the sound transformer mechanism.

The technique of "reconstructive tympanoplasty" has been improved and refined ever since the introduction of operating microscope. The methods of radical and modified radical mastoid operations have not changed for decades except for minor variations. Variety of graft materials being used to restore the dry and functioning ear.

The autologous, homologous, allograft, synthetic materials as plastics, ceramics, hydroxyapatite, gold and recently introduced titanium being used in reconstructive tympano-plasty. But still these grafts have not proved their universal acceptability except the autologous grafts (cartilage, ossicles, fascia). The functioning and survival of each graft material varies as each one has certain advantages and disadvantages and technical problems during and after middle ear reconstruction.

The use of cartilage in middle ear surgery is not a new concept and has been recommended on a limited basis to manage retraction pockets for many years, and more recently it has been used in reconstruction of tympanic membrane recurrent perforations, atelactasis and cholesteatoma pockets. It is naturally thicker and stiffer than fascia, easy to introduce in place and it has less shrinkage and displacement. The tragal cartilage-perichondrium composite graft is an ideal material for posterior canal wall, lateral attic wall and annular reconstruction.

Cartilage is the grafting material of choice in advanced disorders of the middle ear while the indications for its routine use remain controversial due to the possible detrimental effect on postoperative hearing. Aim of the present study was to report personal experience with "cartilage tympanoplasty." The study focused on 600 cases of varied middle ear pathology of safe and unsafe types. In adult patients (450 primary procedures and 150 revisions from January 1980 to June 2010), mean postoperative follow-up was 60 months (range 1–60). The following parameters were evaluated: graft take, change between the pre- and postoperative pure-tone average air-bone gap (PTA-ABG), postoperative complications. Graft take was 99.3% and there were no immediate postoperative complications. The overall average preoperative pure-tone average air-bone gap was 43.79 ± 7.07 dB, whereas the postoperative (3 year after surgery) pure-tone average air-bone gap was 10.43 ±5.25 dB (p <0.0001). Statistically significant improvement was observed up to 5 years after surgery. This study reveals that cartilage tympanoplasty is a reliable technique, in fact it has a high degree of graft take and hearing results are satisfactory. Furthermore, the cartilage is a satisfactory grafting material because it is easily accessible, easy to adopt, resistant to negative middle ear pressures, stable, elastic, well tolerated by the middle ear, resistant to resorption. Therefore, we recommend its use in middle ear reconstruction in which the functional outcome is more essential.

The overall graft take rate of 94 to 96% suggests that cartilage tympanoplasty is a reliable technique, which is in agreement with the results of other authors. In fact, the cartilage is nourished mostly by diffusion and becomes well incorporated in the tympanic membrane. The thickness of the cartilage creates stiffness that is more resistant than the fascia to the anatomic deformation caused by negative middle ear pressure, thus improving long-term integrity.

We might anticipate a significant conductive hearing loss with cartilage owing to its thickness and rigidity. The thickness and rigidity could be reduced by using cartilage slicer, taking 0.5 mm, 1 mm or 2 mm thickness graft material for reconstruction which will improve the hearing results.

The tragal cartilage is typically slightly less than 1 mm thick and, therefore, is used as a full-thickness graft. Using the Doppler interferometer, Zahnert suggested a slight acoustic benefit by thinning the cartilage to 0.5 mm, but this advantage is offset by the curling of the graft. Therefore, since our hearing results have been good, we recommend full-thickness grafts for cartilage reconstruction of the eardrum. The sliced cartilage which are thin could be used in palisade tympanoplasty and attic and posterior canal wall reconstruction.

GOODHILL STUDY

Goodhill in 1964 described the use of the tragal cartilage for ossicular and tympanic reconstruction. Since then several studies have been published describing the use of perichondrium and cartilage in reconstructive tympanoplasty with excellent hearing results. Several studies proved that the hearing results with cartilage to be no different than those for fascia. Cartilage has shown promise as a graft material to close perforations in the tympanic membrane (TM), particularly in cases of advanced middle ear pathology. Although it is similar to fascia, its more rigid quality tends to resist resorption and retraction TM. Because little has been reported in the literature comparing hearing results using cartilage with results using other grafting materials. The retrospective study was conducted to compare the hearing results of patients with cartilage tympanoplasty with fascia. No significant difference was found in the results.

JOHN L DORNHOFFER STUDY

Cartilage has shown promise as a graft material to close perforations in the tympanic membrane (TM), particularly in cases of advanced middle ear pathology. Although it is similar to fascia, its more rigid quality tends to resist resorption and retraction. However, it is this rigid quality that has led many to anticipate a significant conductive hearing loss when using cartilage to reconstruct the middle ear pathology. The average pre- and postoperative pure-tone average air-bone gap (PTA-ABG) was 21.1 dB and 6.8 dB for the cartilage group and 17.9 dB and 7.7 dB for the perichondrium group, respectively. These gains in hearing were statistically significant (P <0.001 in each case), but there was no statistically significant difference in hearing results between the two groups. Analysis of the PTA-ABG as a function of percentage of TM reconstructed showed no statistically significant difference in hearing results due to percentage of cartilage used. These results indicate that cartilage tympanoplasty offers the possibility of a rigorous TM reconstruction with excellent postoperative hearing results.

MIRKO TOS STUDY

Professor Mirko Tos, one of the world's most famous and influential otologists, deals with the application of autogeneous cartilage, harvested from the concha or the tragus, for middle ear reconstructions. Because of the perceived benefits of using cartilage in tympanic membrane and attic reconstruction, this surgical method, called cartilage tympanoplasty, has become increasingly popular, and is now an established procedure in otosurgical practice. Results of surgery illustrate eventual functional differences between the various methods with the aim to promote the basic and clinical research in cartilage tympanoplasty. The main goal of this monograph is to highlight the different methods and techniques and demonstrate the surgical procedures for better understanding. Experienced otosurgeons may also benefit from this monograph.

In this monograph, author has exclusively used the perichondrium-cartilage composite island graft, butterfly graft, the palisade grafts, and schield graft with some technical modifications which have given consistent good results in middle ear reconstruction. In addition, total perichondrium graft with entire tragal cartilage is routinely used in reconstructing old radical cavities. In ossiculoplasty, the cartilage is widely used as interposition material in type II and type III tympanoplasty. Autogenous tragal cartilage plates are widely used for reconstructing attic wall defects in canal wall up mastoidectomy techniques or for reconstructing the entire ear canal in canal wall down mastoidectomy techniques. The cartilage plates technique has prevented recurrent retractions, cholesteatoma and adhesions. This study has excluded children group of less than 10 years in middle ear reconstruction because cartilage is not a good material for achieving good results since in the long run it tends to wrap and is completely resorbed. It is not clear whether it is due to recurrent otitis media or unstable upper respiratory tract.

The author has presented his work on cartilage and perichondrium reconstruction in various middle ear pathologies for over three and half decades at KEM Hospital, Pune, and concluded that cartilage is an ideal graft material for reconstructive tympanoplasty. The results are compatible with fascia graft. The review of literature also reveals that the cartilage is a universally accepted graft material in middle ear reconstruction.

In view of this, the author strongly recommends the **cartilage-perichondrium graft** as a choice graft for reconstructive tympanoplasty. Above all it is most cost-effective for patients. The hearing improvement within 15 dB of BC has become almost a standard criterion for the analysis of surgical success.

Historical Overview

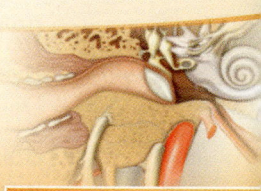

2

Reconstructive ear surgery has undergone many phases from the crude ancient techniques to the modern era of sophisticated micro-ear surgery. Each phase had surgeons who were always in search for an ideal reconstructive material—**The Graft**.

1640 : **Banzar**

Made the first attempt to reconstruct and repair the eardrum using pig's bladder membrane.

1841 : **Yearsley**

Used a moist cotton ball to improve hearing in a perforated drum; by covering the round window from phase interference.

1853 : **Toynbee**

Introduced "artificial membrane tympanic", i.e. a rubber disc with silver wire.

1878 : **Berthold**

Did the first myringoplasty using thick skin graft.

1887 : **Blake**

Recommended the use of paper patch to close the eardrum perforation.

1889 : **Korner**

First suggested that in certain cases of chronic otitis media, the tympanic membrane and ossicles could be left in place during the radical operations, thus preserving good hearing.

1991 : **Nylen**
Developed operating microscope (mono-ocular).

1922 : **Holmgren**
Introduced binocular microscope.

1935 : **Fleming**
Discovered penicillin introducing the antibiotics era, therefore, improving the results with various graft materials.

1951 : **Zollner**
1952 : **Wullestein**
Introduced the concept of tympanoplasty (grafting the middle ear reconstruction). Steps were taken to improve rather than preserve hearing.

1953 : **Wullestein**
Introduced the term "tympanoplasty"—also introduced the use of operating microscope which greatly enchanced the management of pathology.

1958 : **Heermann J et al.**
First used temporal fasica for the repair of the eardrum.

1959 : **Howard House**
First time used polythene in middle ear surgery.

1961 : **Hall and Rytzner**
Pursued the possibility of using a remnants of the patient's own ossicles to create a sound transformed mechanism.

1962 : **Jansen**
Recommended use of homografts septal cartilage.

1962 : **Harris & Goodhill**
First time used autograft tragal cartilage and proved that it was a satisfactory material for ossicular chain reconstruction.

1965 : William House

Used homograft incus for ossicular reconstruction.

1966 : Jules Waltner

Described a new technique in tympanoplasty by using thin strip of tragal cartilage and corrected defects like loss of long process of incus, total loss of incus, absent incus and malleus. Follow-up showed encouraging results, a complete closure of A-B gap in nine out of ten patients.

1966 : Brackman

In thirty cases where the stapedial crura were absent, the use of a perichondrium–tragal cartilage unit (T-shaped) creating a natural columella gave good results.

1967 : Victor Goodhill

Concluded that perichondrium and cartilage obtained from the tragus provide viable autograft materials for tympanoplastic reconstruction. He limited the use in type I and type III tympanoplasty.

1967 : Irwin Harris and Victor Goodhill

Described various applications of tragal cartilage graft techniques in middle ear surgery like in problems of stapedectomy, poststapedectomy incudostapedial necrosis, and total ossicular necrosis with tympanic membrane perforation.

Results were excellent three years postoperatively.

1967 : MC Shea and ME Glasscock

Reported 172 cases of tympanoplasty with cartilage prosthesis. They had employed three basic shapes of cartilage, viz a long thin shaft with notched head, a T-shaped piece to fit over the head of stapes. Though they came across various minor and major problems, they had encouraging results, viz. 65% A-B gap closure to within 20 dB.

1973 : Claus Jansen

Stated that autologous conchal or tragal cartilage in the form of a ring prosthesis used to raise the level of stapes was much better than auto-ossicles because the cartilage could be cut more accurately and shaped more quickly than others. To minimize immunologic and for storage purpose, the cartilage was preserved in a rapidly hardening acrylic palaces.

Histological examination showed no change in the cartilage structure even after 7 years.

1973 : Jack Pulec and James Sheehy

Described various techniques of ossicular chain reconstruction using auto-ossicle grafts, homografts, and cartilage grafts. They showed that, cartilage struts do not become fixed by bone. Even when kept under considerable tension against the tympanic membrane, the cartilage does not seem to extrude, and a more firm contact with the mobile foot-plate is thus assured.

1975 : Andrew Don and Fred Linthicum

Autograft tragal cartilages from revision tympanoplasty were examined with histologic and histochemical stains. The implanted cartilages were without significant inflammatory reaction or evidence of resorption and have been well tolerated in the middle ear space.

1978 : Altenau and Sheehy

Reported 564 tympanoplasties using tragal cartilage as an ossicular substitute. Cartilage strut with perichondrium was used under tension between tympanic membrane and stapes foot-plate. Cartilage block was used between malleus and head of stapes. This could simultaneously block attic defects and prevent posterior retraction pockets. Various causes of failure, like short cartilage, displaced cartilage (medial and/or lateral ends), fibrosis around cartilage, cartilage extrusion, were identified and rectified.

They also suggested that plastic prosthesis (TORP and PORP) with cartilage interposed between the prosthesis and tympanic membrane appear to be more effective than cartilage alone.

1978 : Abraham Eviatar

137 tympanoplasties with ossicular reconstruction using tragal cartilage were described with good post-operative results.

1981 : E Steinbach and A Pusalkar

Studied long-term histological changes in the cartilage after doing ossicular reconstruction using tragal cartilage. 52 cases were studied. Various macroscopic changes like change in shape (irregularity, softening, necrosis) and microscopic changes like changes in the appearance of chondrocytes which lose their paired character and become irregular. In some, the cartilage was replaced by firbosis while in some cartilages, lacunae were found indicating resorptive process. This study clearly demonstrated the main causes of failure in ossicular reconstruction by tragal cartilage.

1986 : Diran O Mikaelian

Described a one stage reconstruction of tympanic membrane and the ossicular chain using a composite graft of tragal perichondrium with cartilage (Type III tympanoplasty). He did all operations under local anaesthesia.

1989 : Mangham CA and East CA

Compared the composite tragal perichondrium and cartilage autografts vs cartilage or bone paste grafts in tympanoplasty and achieved good results with composite grafts after two years follow-up.

1992 : Heerman J

Tympanomastoid reconstruction using tragal perichondrium and conchal palisade cartilage.

1982 : Mirko Tos
Modifications of combined approach tympanoplasty in attic cholesteatoma.
Classifications and methods of cartilage tympanoplasty, tympanoplasty in missing malleous handle.

2006 : John L Dornhoffer
Cartilage tympanoplasty
Cartilage schield T-tube in cartilageplasty

Surgical Anatomy of the Middle Ear

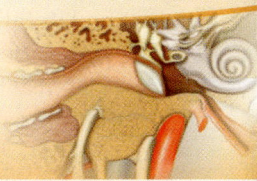

3

The middle ear cleft includes the tympanum (middle ear cavity proper), the Eustachean tube, and the mastoid air cell system. The tympanic cavity is an air-filled irregular space contained within the temporal bone. It also contains the three auditory ossicles (malleus, incus and stapes) along with their attached muscles. For the purpose of description, the tympanic cavity may be considered as a box with four walls, a roof and a floor. The corners of this hypothetical box are not sharp.

LATERAL WALL

The lateral wall of the tympanum/middle ear is partly bony and partly membranous. The central portion of the lateral wall is formed by the tympanic membrane, while above and below the tympanic membrane there is bone, forming the outer lateral walls of the epitympanum (attic) and hypotympanum, respectively. The lateral wall of the epitympanum (attic) also includes that part of the tympanic membrane lying above the anterior and posterior malleolar folds—this portion of the ear-drum is also known as pars flaccida. This portion of the tympanic membrane lacks the middle fibrous layer, hence the name. The lateral attic wall (bony portion) is wedge-shaped, its lower portion is also called the outer attic wall (scutum). Scutum actually means sheild in Latin. This bony portion is thin and its lateral surface forms the superior portion of the deep portion of the external meatus.

Three openings are present in the bone of the medial surface of the lateral wall of the tympanic cavity. The first opening is the posterior canaliculus for the chorda tympani. This opening is situated at the junction between the lateral and posterior walls of the tympanic cavity. This opening is usually present at the level of the upper end of the handle of the malleus. This opening leads to the bony canal which descends through the posterior wall of the tympanic cavity. Since chorda tympani traverses this canal, it is also known as the canal for chorda tympani nerve. This canal also contains a branch from the stylomastoid artery which usually accompanies the chorda tympani.

The second opening is the petrotympanic (Glaserian) fissure. This fissure opens anteriorly just above the attachment of the tympanic membrane. This opening is infact a small slit about 2 mm long. It receives the anterior malleolar ligament. It also transmits the anterior tympanic branch of the maxillary artery to the tympanic cavity.

The third is the canal of Hugier. It lies medial to the Glaserian fissure. The chorda tympani enters through this.

ROOF

The roof of the middle ear cavity is formed by the tegmen tympani. It is this tegmen tympani which separates the middle ear cavity from the dura of the middle cranial fossa. This tegmen tympani is formed in part by the petrous portion of the temporal bone, and the squamous portion of the temporal bone. The suture line between these two components is known as the petrosquamous suture line. This suture line is unossified in the young, and does not close until adult life is reached. Through this suture, veins from the middle ear may pass to the superior petrosal sinus.

FLOOR

The floor is much narrow. Infact it is narrower than the roof of the middle ear cavity. This portion of the middle ear cavity lies in close relationship with the jugular bulb. The middle ear cavity is separated from the jugular bulb by a thin piece of bone. Rarely, the floor may be deficient and the jugular bulb in these patients is separated from the middle ear cavity only by fibrous tissue and mucous membrane. At the junction of the floor and the medial wall of the middle ear, there is a small opening which allows the entry of tympanic branch of glossopharyngeal nerve to pass into the middle ear. This nerve takes an important part in the formation of tympanic plexus.

ANTERIOR WALL

The anterior wall of the tympanic cavity is very narrow. This is because the medial and lateral walls converge anteriorly. The anterior wall can be divided into two portions; the upper and lower portions. The lower portion of the anterior wall is larger than the upper portion. It has a thin plate of bone which separates this portion from the internal carotid artery as it enters the skull. This plate has two openings for the caroticotympanic nerves. The upper opening transmits the superior caroticotympanic nerve and the inferior opening transmits the inferior caroticotympanic nerve. It is through these nerves that sympathetic nerves reach the tympanic plexus. The upper smaller part of the anterior wall has two tunnels placed one below the other. The upper tunnel transmits the tensor tympani muscle, and the lower tunnel transmits the bony portion of the eustachean tube.

MEDIAL WALL

The medial wall separates the middle ear from the inner ear. The most prominent portion of the medial wall of the middle ear cavity is the promontory. It is a rounded projection occupying most of the central portion of the medial wall of the middle ear. This projection is raised by the underlying basal turn of the cochlea. The promontory has numerous small grooves on its surface. These grooves contain the tympanic plexus of nerves. Behind and above the promontory is the oval window (fenestra vestibuli). This is a oval-shaped opening connecting the tympanic cavity with the vestibule. In life, this is closed by the foot plate of stapes and its surrounding annular ligament. The long axis of the fenestra vestibuli is horizontal. Its inferior border is concave. The size of the oval window varies, but on an average it is 3.25 mm long and 1.75 mm wide. Above this fenestra vestibuli is the canal for facial nerver (horizontal portion) and below lies the promontory. Hence the fenestra vestibuli lies at the bottom of a depression also known as fossula that can be of varying depths depending on the position of the facial nerve and the prominence of the promontory

The fenestra cochlea (round window) lies just below and behind the oval window. It is closed in life by a membrane known as the round window membrane (secondary tympanic membrane). The secondary tympanic membrane appears to be divided into an anterior and posterior portions by the presence of a transverse thickening. The diameter of the round window membrane is between 1.8 and 2.3 mm. It is made up of three layers; the outer mucosal, middle fibrous and an inner endothelial layer. The membrane of the fenestra cochleae does not lie at the end of the scala tympani but forms part of its floor.

The ampulla of the posterior semicircular canal is the closest vestibular structure to this membrane. The nerve supplying the ampulla of the posterior semicirular canal (singular nerve) lies close to this secondary tympanic membrane. The secondary tympanic membrane forms a landmark for the position of the singular nerve. This is useful during surgical procedures like singular neurectomy for treatment of intractable vertigo.

These two windows (oval and round) are separated by the posterior extension of the promontory. This is known as the subiculum. Rarely a spicule of bone arises from the promontory above the subiculum and runs to the pyramid on the posterior wall of the middle ear cavity. This spicule of bone is known as the ponticulus. The round window faces inferiorly and a little posteriorly, lying completely under the cover of the promontory and hence usually is difficult to visualise. The round window niche is usually trianglular in shape, having anterior, posterosuperior and posteroinferior walls. The posterosuperior and posteroinferior walls meet posteriorly leading on to the sinus tympani. This sinus tympani is a difficult area to visualise.

Cholesteatoma may lurk in this area making it difficult to remove. This is one of the commonest causes of cholesteatoma recurrence after mastoidectomy. Small mirrors known as the zinne mirror can be used to visualise this area indirectly. Since sinus tympani lies under the pyramid, removal of the pyramid during surgery will bring the sinus tympani area into view. The facial nerve canal is another important anatomical structure present in this wall. This nerve runs above the promontory and fenestra vestibuli in an anteroposterior direction. The canal may occasionally be deficient leaving an exposed facial nerve. This is a dangerous anatomical variant because this nerve can easily be traumatised during any surgical procedures in the middle ear cavity. Even infections of the middle ear mucosa can cause facial nerve palsy in patients with an exposed facial nerve. The anterior end of the facial nerve canal is marked by the presence of a bony process known as processus cochleariformis. This curved projection of bone is concave anteriorly and it houses the tendon of the tensor tympani muscle as it turns laterally to the handle of the malleus. Behind the fenestra vestibuli, the facial nerve turns inferiorly to begin its descent in the posterior wall of the tympanic cavity.

The region above the level of the facial nerve canal forms the medial wall of the epitympanum or attic. The dome of the lateral semicircular canal extends a little lateral to the facial canal and is the major feature of the posterior portion of the epitympanum. In well-pneumatised bones, this dome of the lateral canal can be very prominent

POSTERIOR WALL

The posterior wall of the middle ear is wider above than below. In its upper part, it has an important opening known as the aditus. This aditus helps the middle ear to communicate with the mastoid air cell system. Aditus is a large irregular opening connecting the mastoid antrum to the middle ear cavity. Below the aditus is a small depression known as the fossa incudis. Fossa incudis houses the short process of the incus. Below the fossa incudis lies the pyramid.

Pyramid is a small conical projection which is hollow and its apex pointing anteriorly. It contains the stapedius muscle, the tendon of which passes forwards to insert into the neck of the stapes. The canal within the promontory curves downwards and backwards to join the descending portion of the facial nerve canal. Between the promontory and the tympanic annulus is the facial recess.

The facial recess is bounded medially by the facial nerve and laterally by the tympanic annulus. Running through the wall between the two with varying degrees of obliquity is the chorda tympani nerve. This nerve always runs medial to the tympanic membrane. Drilling over the facial recess area between the facial nerve and the annulus in the angle formed by the chorda tympani nerve can lead into the middle ear cavity. This surgical approach to the middle ear cavity through this area is known as the facial recess approach. This approcah is suitable for surgeries involving the round window niche like placement of electrodes during cochlear implant procedures. Hypotympanum can also be approached through this approach.

CONTENTS OF THE MIDDLE EAR

The most important content of the middle ear is air. The air flows into the middle ear through a patent eustachean tube. The other contents are chain of three ossicles which help in sound transmission; the malleus, incus and stapes. Two muscles, chorda tympani nerve and the tympanic plexus of nerves.

Malleus

This bone is shaped like a hammer hence the name. This is the largest of the three ossicles of the middle ear cavity. It has a head, neck and three processes arising from below the neck. The overall length of the malleus ranges between 7.5 and 9 mm. Its head lies in the attic region of the middle ear effectively dividing the attic into an anterior portion and a posterior one. The anterior portion lies anterior to the handle of the malleus, while the posterior portion lies behind the handle of the malleus.

During surgical procedures for attic cholesteatoma, clipping of this head will improve the exposure in the attic region. The head of the malleus on its posteromedial surface has an elongated saddle-shaped cartilage covered facet for articulation with the incus. This articular surface is constricted near its

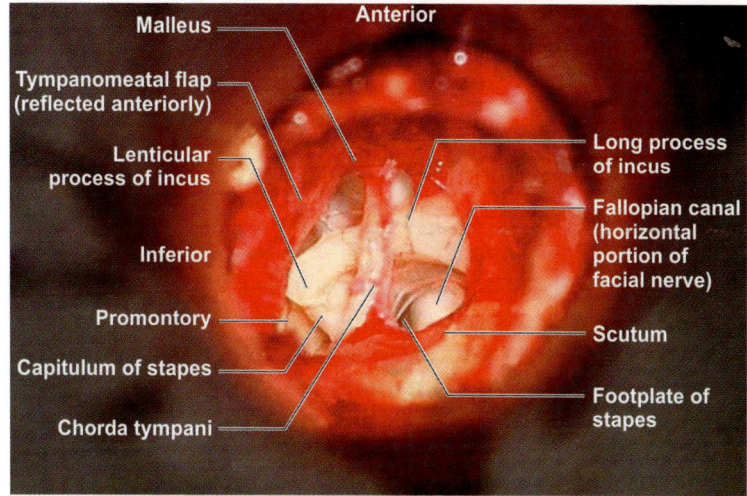

Fig. 3.1. Left middle ear—surgeon's view

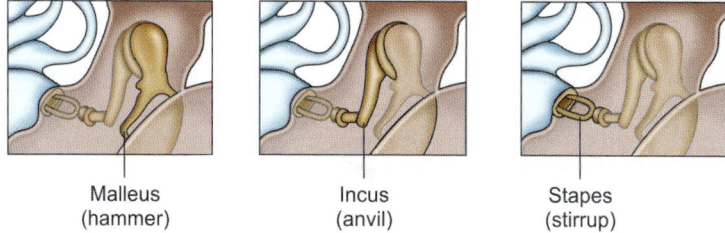

Fig. 3.2. Middle ear bones

middle dividing the articular facet into a larger superior and a smaller inferior portions. The inferior portion of the articular facet lies at right angles to that of the superior portion.

This projecting lower portion is also known as the cog or spur of the malleus. Below the neck the bone broadens and gives rise to the following: the anterior process from which a slender anterior ligament arises to insert into the petrotympanic fissure; the lateral process which receives the anterior and posterior malleolar folds from the annulus tympanicum, and the handle which runs downwards, medially and slightly backwards between the mucous and fibrous layers of the tympanic membrane. On the deep medial surface of the handle, there is a small projection into which the tendon of the tensor tympani muscle inserts. Additionally, the malleus is supported by the superior ligament which runs from the head to the tegmen tympani.

Incus

This bone is shaped like an anvil. It articulates with the malleus and has a body and two processes. The body lies in the attic and has a cartilage covered articular facet corresponding to that of the malleus. The short process projects backwards from the body to lie in the fossa incudis. It is in fact attached to the fossa incudis by a short ligament. The long process of the incus descends into the mesotympanum behind and medial to the handle of the malleus. At its tip, there is a small medially directed lenticular process which articulates with the stapes. The long process of the incus has precarious blood supply. This portion of the incus is prone for undergoing necrosis in disease conditions.

Stapes

The stapes consists of a head, neck, two crura and a base (footplate). The head of the stapes points laterally and has a small cartilage covered depression for articulation with the lenticular process of the incus. The tendon of the stapedius muscle attaches to the posterior part of the neck and the upper part of the posterior crura. The neck of the stapes gives rise to two crura, the anterior crura is thinner and less curved than the posterior crura. The two crura join the footplate which closes the oval window during life. The average dimensions of the footplate is 3 × 1.4 mm. The long axis of the footplate is almost horizontal, with the posterior end being slightly lower than the anterior.

MUSCLES OF MIDDLE EAR

Stapedius Muscle

This muscle arises from the walls of the concial cavity within the pyramid. A slender tendon emerges from the apex of the pyramid and inserts into the stapes. This muscle is supplied by a small branch from the facial nerve. The stapedial tendon is inserted into the neck of the stapes. On contraction, this muscle rocks the stapes backwards holding it firm against the annular ligament preventing excessive transmission of sound into the inner ear. This muscle has a protective role to play. It protects the inner ear from insults caused by loud noise. Patients with facial nerve palsy have hyperacusis because of lack of action of this muscle.

Tensor Tympani Muscle

This long slender muscle arises from the walls of the bony canal which lie above the canal for the eustachean tube. Parts of the muscle also arise from the cartilagenous portion of the eustachean tube and the greater wing of sphenoid. From these origins, the muscle passes backwards into the tympanic cavity lying on the medial wall of the middle ear just below the level of the facial nerve. The bony covering of the canal is often deficient in its tympanic segment where the muscle is replaced by its tendon. This tendon enters the processus cochleariformis, turns at right angles inserting into the medial aspect of the upper end of the handle of the malleus. This muscle is supplied by the mandibular nerve by way of a branch from the medial pterygoid nerve, which passes through the otic ganglion without synapsing. This muscle tenses the tympanic membrane by holding the handle of the malleus thus helping the middle ear in better sound perception.

Chorda Tympani Nerve

This is a branch of the facial nerve. It enters the middle ear cavity through the posterior canaliculus which is present at the junction of the lateral and posterior walls. It runs across the medial surface of the tympanic membrane between the mucosal and fibrous layers passes medial to the upper portion of the handle of the malleus. Here it lies above the tendon of the tensor tympani muscle, continues forwards and leaves by way of the anterior canaliculus placed within the petrotympanic fissure. It joins the lingual branch of the V nerve with which it is distributed to the anterior one-third of the tongue.

Tympanic Plexus

It is found over the promontory. It is formed by the tympanic branch of the glossopharyngeal nerve, caroticotympanic nerves which supplies the sympathetic component. The tympanic plexus provides the following branches:

1. Branches to the mucous membrane lining the tympanic cavity, eustachean tube, mastoid antrum and its air cells.
2. A branch joining the greater superficial petrosal nerve.
3. The lesser superficial petrosal nerve, which contains all the parasympathetic fibers of the IX nerve. This nerve leaves the middle ear through a small canal below the tensor tympani muscle where it receives parasympathetic fibres from the VII nerve by way of a branch from the geniculate ganglion. The full nerve passes through the temporal bone to emerge lateral to the greater superficial petrosal nerve on the floor of the middle cranial fossa, outside the dura. It then passes through the foramen ovale with the mandibular nerve and accessory meningeal artery to the otic ganglion. Post-ganglionic fibres from the otic ganglion supply secretomotor fibres to the parotid gland by way of the auriculotemporal nerve.

The mucosal lining of the middle ear cavity varies according to the location. The attic or the epitympanum is lined by pavement epithelium, while the middle ear proper is lined by cuboidal epithelium and the hypotympanum is lined by ciliated columnar epithelium.

Physiological Principles in Middle Ear Transformer Mechanism

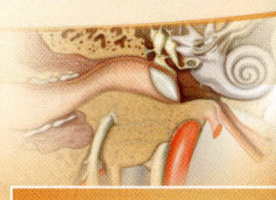

4

The process of hearing begins with the occurrence of a sound. Sound is initiated when an event moves and causes a motion or vibration in air. When this air movement stimulates the ear, a sound is heard.

In the human ear, a sound wave is transmitted through four separate media along the auditory system before a sound is perceived (Fig. 4.1): in the outer ear—air, in the middle ear—mechanical, in the inner ear—liquid, and to the brain—neural.

2. The auditory ossicles vibrate and the footplate of the stapes moves at the oval window

3. Movement of the oval window causes the fluid inside the scala vestibuli and scala tympani to move

4. Fluid movement against the cachlear duct sets off nerve impulses, which are carried to the brain via the cochlear nerve

1. Sound vibrations strike the eardrum

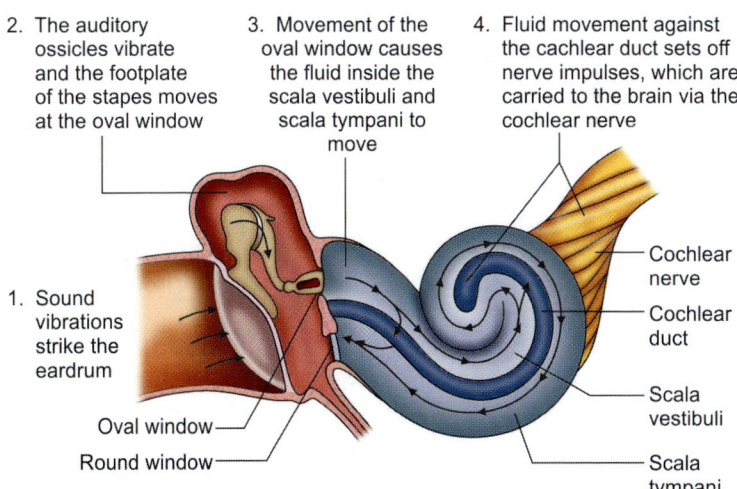

Cochlear nerve

Cochlear duct

Scala vestibuli

Scala tympani

Oval window

Round window

Fig. 4.1. Transformer machanism of sound conduction

23

Sound Transmission through Outer Ear

Air transmitted sound waves are directed toward the delicate hearing mechanisms with the help of the outer ear, first by the pinna, which gently funnels sound waves into the ear canal, then by the ear canal.

Sound Transmission through Middle Ear

The air movement strikes the tympanic membrane, the tympanic membrane or eardrum moves. At this point, the energy generated through a sound wave is transferred from a medium of air to that which is solid in the middle ear. The ossicular chain of the middle ear connects to the eardrum via the malleus, so that any motion of the eardrum sets the three little bones of the ossicular chain into motion.

Sound Transmission through Inner Ear

The ossicular chain transfers energy from a solid medium to the fluid medium of the inner ear via the stapes. The stapes is attached to the oval window. Movement of the oval window creates motion in the cochlear fluid and along the basilar membrane. Motion along the basilar membrane excites frequency specific areas of the organ of Corti, which in turn stimulates a series of nerve endings.

Sound Transmission to Brain

With the initiation of the nerve impulses, another change in medium occurs: from fluid to neural. Nerve impulses are relayed through the VIII CN, through various nuclei along the auditory pathway to areas to the brain. It is the brain that interprets the neural impulses and creates a thought, picture, or other recognized symbol.

An understanding of the physiology of the middle ear begins from the oval and round windows. In order that vibratory movements may take place at the cochlear partition in response to the sound energy, it is essential that the two windows are free to vibrate reciprocally, i.e. in the opposite phase. This will not occur, if both the windows are exposed to the same wavefront, under the same functional conditions as in this situation to-and-fro movement of the cochlear fluids could result.

In the intact ear, sound energy is transmitted through the tympanic membrane and ossicular chain to the oval window. A very small fraction of the total energy reaches the round window by air conduction across the tympanic cavity and this in phase pressure is too weak to interfere significantly, the reciprocal pressure on the round window reaching it by the cochlear fluid and oval window route. Thus, the intact tympanic membrane protects the round window and feeds the ossicular chain and oval window.

Current views state that the round window does not lie in the direct sound pathway to the cochlea but it functions as reliving point. Its mobility is as essential to normal hearing as that of any part of vibrating system. The malleus and incus vibrate as a combined unit rocking on a linear axis, which runs from the anterior ligament of the malleus to the attachment of the short process of the incus in the fossa incudis. When reciprocating movements of the conducting system take place, the mass of the body of the incus and the head and neck of the malleus lying above this axis serve to balance the mass of the drum head, malleus handle, long process of incus and stapes lying below it.

The movement of the stapes is more complex, with sounds of moderate intensity; the anterior end of the footplate oscillates with greater amplitude than the posterior end. This is because the fibres of the annular ligament are longer at the anterior end than those at the posterior end.

With sounds of high intensity, the mode of action changes and a side-to-side rocking movement is seen about an axis running longitudinally though the length of the footplate. Obviously, the displacement of inner ear fluid volume will be less in the second vibratory mode than in the first. These alternative stapedial mechanisms constitute a protective arrangement for minimizing too violent a stimulation of the inner ear. In the intact middle ear, impedance matching is brought about so that which amplitude is greatly reduced at the oval window, is increased in the same proportion.

This mechanism depends on **ossicular chain lever ratio.** The malleus and incus jointly act as a lever, pivoting upon the axis of rotation. The malleolar arm is longer than the incudated arm in the ratio 1.3:1.

The Areal Ratio of Tympanic Membrane and Oval Window

There is a hydraulic effect between these two structures, increasing the forces of vibration at the oval window undiminished; the increase in the force will be in the same ratio as the ratio between the effective area of the tympanic membrane and the oval window (the effective area of the tympanic membrane is appreciably lesser than its total area since it is fixed all round the periphery). The effective area of the tympanic membrane is found to be two-thirds of its anatomical area. If the area of the oval window is measured, an effective area ratio between these two structures of 14:1 is obtained. The overall ratio for the middle ear is the product of the ossicular chain lever ratio and the area between the tympanic membrane and oval window. This is approximately 18.3. By definition the impedance transformation ratio is the square of this figure and is, therefore, 336. The ratio of acoustic impedance of air and water is 3880, so it becomes evident that the impedance matching due to middle ear, although very substantial is theoretically, at lease, less than ideally required.

Surgical Pathology

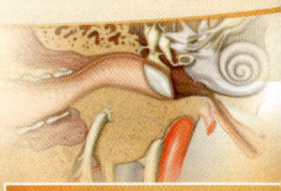

5

Chronic suppurative otitis media (CSOM) has traditionally been classified into safe ear disease and unsafe ear disease. Safe ear disease, sometimes called tubotympanic disease, is characterized as a central perforation of the pars tensa with the inflammatory process affecting the mucosa of the middle ear cleft. Unsafe ear disease, sometimes called atticoantral disease, is typified by a marginal perforation of the posterosuperior pars tensa or pars flaccida. Cholesteatoma is frequently present in CSOM with posterosuperior perforations. Partially due to induced bony erosion and secondary infection, cholesteatomas can lead to potentially devastating sequelae. Admittedly, all cases of CSOM, including those described above as safe, can be associated with serious intracranial complications. Therefore, the term safe does not adequately categorize any cases of CSOM.

CSOM can be more simply divided into mucosal disease and cholesteatoma. Mucosal disease is typified by a bacterial infection of the middle ear cleft with the presence of pus, associated with discharge through a pars tensa perforation, for longer than 3 months. Acquired cholesteatoma, usually arising from the pars flaccida skin, typically involves the epitympanum and the mastoid antrum and, as stated above, can be erosive, causing serious complications.

Eosinophilic otitis media is an intractable middle ear disease associated with bronchial asthma and nasal allergy that sometimes induces deterioration of sensorineural hearing loss. Determined, active eosinophilic inflammation may occur in the entire respiratory tract, including the middle ear, in patients with this disease. EOM often produces a yellow and highly viscous middle ear effusion and can cause symptoms that range from prolonged hearing loss and otorrhoea to sudden

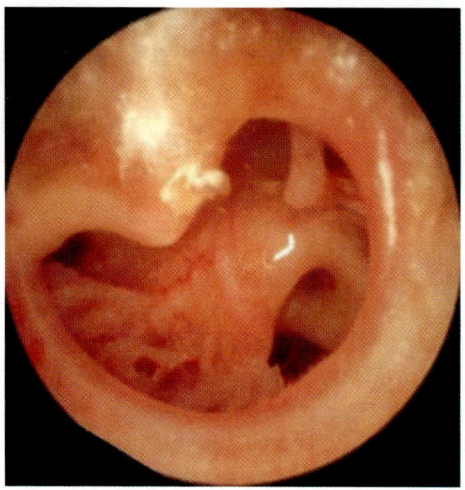

Fig. 5.1. Large central perforation

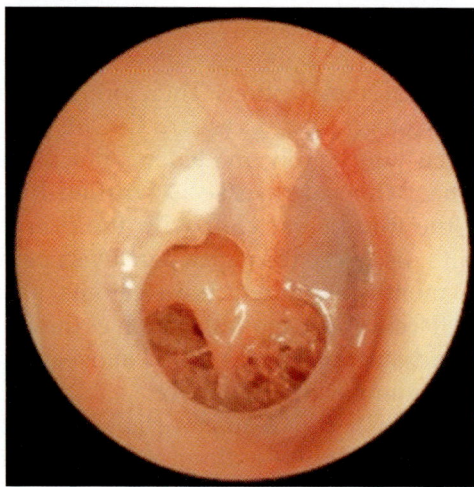

Fig. 5.2. Small central perforation

deafness. The middle ear symptoms are unresponsive to conventional treatments for otitis media and are instead treated with steroids.

Perforation of the drum and ossicular destruction forms an important aspect of chronic otitis media. Both of these can get affected in cases of chronic suppurative otitis media with or without cholesteatoma, and chronic non-suppurative otitis media.

Macroscopically, drum shows evidence of a mechanical defect in the pars tensa or flaccida or there is defect in the ossicles in the form of a destruction of a process, or head or any other part, while the rest of the ossicles are intact, of these may be a total destruction, resulting in a missing ossicle.

Microscopically, there are changes in the epithelium, submucosa and the bony tissue like:

1. Loss of fibrous layer, therefore, thinning the membrane which perforates easily.
2. The simple squamous epithelium undergoes metaplasia to stratified squamous epithelium.
3. There is marked proliferation of granulation tissue.
4. Increased vascularity with thickened walls of blood vessels.
5. Infiltration by round cells macrophages and lymphocytes.
6. There is destruction of the bone adjacent to marrow spaces.
7. It is observed that inflammatory process may be the cause of a defect in tympanic membrane, which gives way easily for the middle ear fluid under tension to escape out side.
8. Hyperaemia and chronic inflammation may be the probable causes of bone resorption, instead of a vascular necrosis which was preciously thought to be the cause of bone destruction, in cases of chronic suppurative otitis media (Sade).
9. Collagenase has been demonstrated in cholesteatoma matrix and macrophages are supposed to be a source of collagenase (Abramson) which is responsible for bone destruction or even the sheer weight of the choesteatoma sac along with its keratin contents, is postulated to cause pressure necrosis and erosion of the ossicles.

10. In adhesive otitis media, adhesive changes may affect tympanic membrane, the middle ear cavity, ossicular chain and the mastoid air cells. Many times, the middle ear cavity is replaced by masses of scar tissue and often there is absorption of bone affecting the ossicular chain.

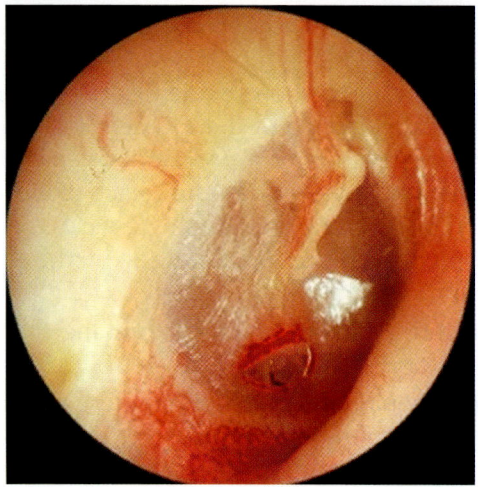

Fig. 5.3. Traumatic perforation

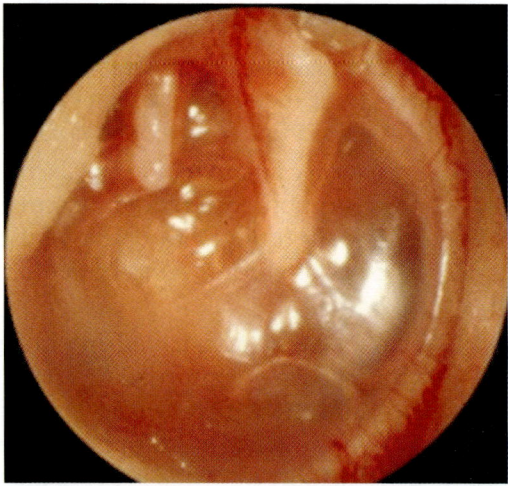

Fig. 5.4. Tympanosclerosis

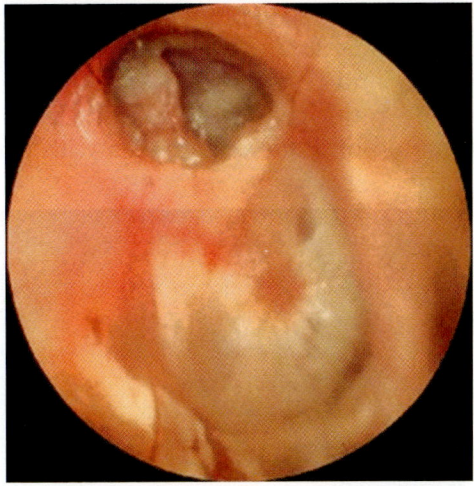

Fig. 5.5. Attic cholesteatoma

In tympanosclerosis, there is a local deposition of plaques of collagen beneath the lining epithelium. Tympanosclerosis is usually seen in the stratum fibrosum of tympanic membrane in middle ear.

PATHOGENESIS IN RE-PERFORATION

Larger perforation is associated with significant lower rate (74%) of success of tympanoplasty. **Success rate is lower in anterior perforation (65%) than posterior perforation (90%).** Presence of middle ear mucosa and contralateral disease is also significant predictors for outcome. A finding of otorrhoea at surgery is a poor prognostic factor for tympanoplasty. Smoking, allergy and resistant infections are associated with worse middle ear status and delayed graft failure. Despite concerns about operating on young children who are prone to otitis media, Albera's study shows that TM closure and re-perforation rates are similar among patients aged less than 18, 18–50, and greater than 50.

The early reperforations were presumably failures in surgery. Less experienced surgeons and inflamed, wet middle ear mucosa during the primary surgery seemed to be the two most important causal factors. Young age at surgery, size and site of the perforation and Eustachian tube function seemed to be of no importance for reperforation. The early reperforations were closed at surgery and remained closed into adulthood. The reasons for late reperforations are less clear; they were presumably caused by acute otitis media with perforation in

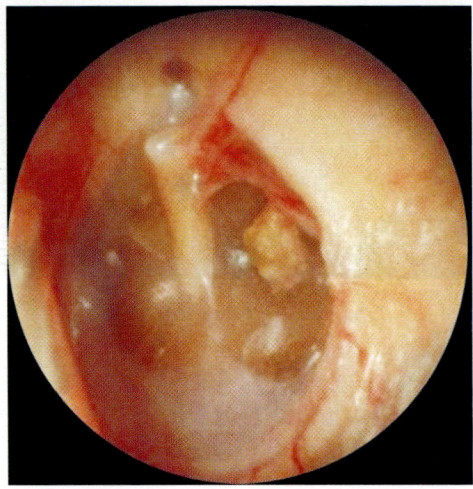

Fig. 5.6. Incudomyringopexy

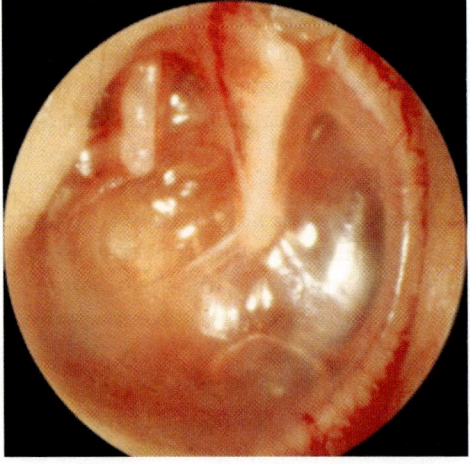

Fig. 5.7. Severe TM atelectasis

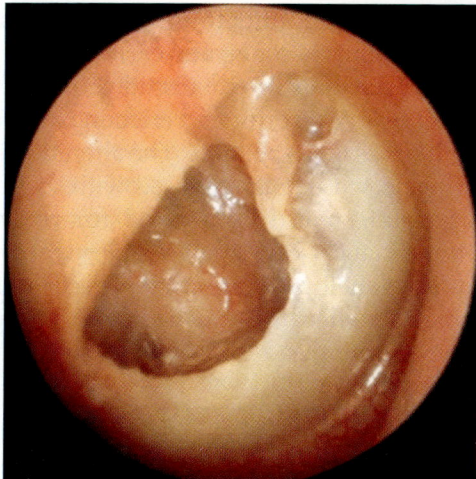

Fig. 5.8. Pars tensa perforation

an atrophic part of the drum, which did not heal. The reperforations were small, but it was possible to close all of them surgically, if the patients wanted to be reoperated. It is concluded that tympanoplasty, even in young children, is a rewarding option with good and stable results.

HISTOCHEMICAL CONSIDERATIONS IN CARTILAGE AUTOGRAFTS

The use of cartilage in tympanoplasty was introduced in early 1963 by Jansan. Several authors have described the histological changes in intratympanic cartilage struts as well as long-term clinical results (Shea and Glossclock in 1967, Smith and Kerr 1970, Smyth et al 1975, Steinback and Pusalkar 1985).

Histochemical examination of lactic dehydrogenase enzyme activity was used to detect the effect of certain factors on the viability of cartilage autografts in the middle ear. The study shows that the presence of perichondrium on both sides of the strut and placing the lateral end of the strut increase the chance of survival of chondrocytes. On the other hand, middle ear infection has a very bad effect on the viability of chondrocytes. The length of the strut and the presence of silastic film in the middle ear have been found to be unimportant as far as the survival of the graft is concerned.

The cartilage graft implanted subcutaneously can be used reliably without fear of resorption. Perichondrium on one side must be kept intact as far as possible. The alteration in the shape of cartilage is expected but can be used with scoring so that a thin cartilage plate could be grafted for reconstruction. Perichondrium enhances cartilage graft survival and seems to act as a protecting shell preventing the direct exposure of the graft to the notorious effects of local mediators of wound healing enviornment that might lead to cartilage resorption.

SCANNING ELECTRON MICROSCOPE

The preimplanted control cartilage grafts showed cartilagenous plates with perichondrium on both sides. Numerous, closely scanning electron microscope: packed, empty lacunae were seen within the cartilage matrix which appeared homogenous. All

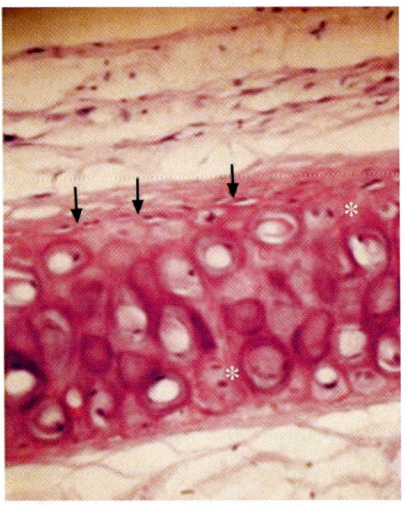

Fig. 5.9. Histochemistry in implanted cartilage autografts: Photomicrograph of the control preimplanted cartilage graft showing normal elastic cartilage with numerous aggregated lacunae containing chondrocytes and moderate amount of matrix in between. The perichondrium appears on both sides with its two layers fibrous (short arrows) and cellular (long arrows).

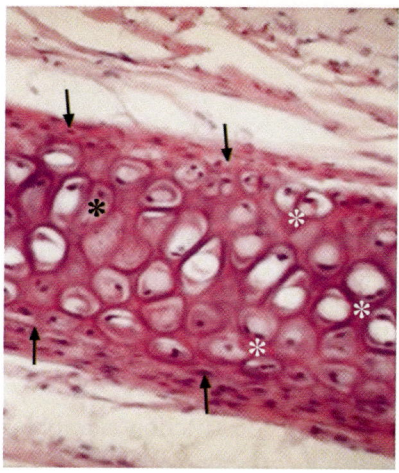

Fig. 5.10. Histochemistry in implanted cartilage autografts: Photomicrograph of a cartilage graft without perichondrium 12 weeks after implantation showing thin cartilage plate with viable chondrocytes inside lacunae

the postimplanted cartilage grafts confirm the previously mentioned gross and light microscopic examination as regard the viability of the cartilage of all grafts 12 weeks after implantation and the absence of either necrotic or fibrous tissue within the grafts. Proliferation of chondroblasts was noticed by the apparent small fusiform lacunae underneath the intact perichondrium in unscored cartilaginous grafts that kept either one side or both sides of perichondrium. There was no evidence for similar cellular proliferation in cartilage grafts denuded from their perichondrium or in scored cartilage grafts. In all examined grafts, the intercellular matrix was intact, moderate in amount and showed no signs of cartilage resorption.

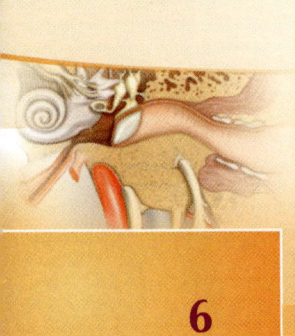

Principles in Cartilage Tympanoplasty

6

The goal of functional reconstruction is to obtain a permanent restoration of hearing. Surgical reconstruction of middle ear transformer mechanism which has been destroyed or impaired due to disease is the essence of tympanoplasty.

1. Complete removal of the disease in same or earlier stage.
2. A conductive hearing loss with a good cochlear reserve as indicated by 30 dB or better bone conduction hearing threshold over speech frequencies.
3. The Eustachain tube function must be normal.
4. Type of ossicular chain defect, condition of individual ossicles and condition of labyrinthine windows should be assessed.
5. Middle ear mucosa should be healthy.

PRINCIPLES

1. To establish communication between intact drum and inner ear fluid, thus restoring middle ear transformer mechanism.
2. To create an air-containing middle ear space with near normal middle ear volume.
3. To achieve mobility of newly formed ossicular chain.

CLASSIFICATION OF TYMPANOPLASTY

Type 1   : Closure of perforation with intact ossicular chain.
Type 2   : Reconstruction of perforated eardrum with the

ossicular reconstruction by interpositioning of various ossicular grafts.

Type 3   : Absent or defective stapedial arch (collumella effect)

Type 4   : Sound protection of round window with cartilage graft.

Type 5A   : Fenestration of lateral semicircular canal.

Type 5B   : Platinectomy (oval window filled with peri-chondrium)

VARIOUS GRAFTS USED FOR RECONSTRUCTIVE EAR SURGERY

(1) Natural and (2) synthetic/biomaterials

1. Natural

Four types of grafts can be defined according to the genetic relationship between donor and host:

1. **Autograft:** Tissue transplanted from one part of the body to another in the same individual, e.g. ossicular bone, cortical bone, cartilage and fascia.

2. **Isograft:** Tissue transplanted between genetically identical individuals, e.g. ossicular bone, cortical bone, cartilage and fascia.

3. **Homograft/allograft:** Tissue transplanted between genetically non-identical members of the same species, e.g. ossicular bone, cortical bone, cartilage and fascia.

4. **Xenograft:** Tissue transplanted between members of different species.

Advantages and Disadvantages

A. Ossicles and cortical bone (auto-/isograft)

Advantages   • Best tolerated.

                  • Lest likely to extrude

Disadvantages   • Displacement

                  • Refixation

                  • Tendency to adhere to surrounding bone.

                  • Atrophy

B. Cartilages—septal/tragal/conchal (auto-/isograft)

Advantages	• Easily available
	• Easily shaped
	• Well tolerated
	• Less extrusion or absorption
Disadvantage	• Lacks stiffness.

C. Fascia—temporalis (auto-/isograft)

Advantages	• Available from the same surgical site.
	• As much as needed can be taken.
	• Consistency is same as that of tympanic membrane.
	• Least likely to extrude.
Disadvantage	• Lacks stiffness so may need a composite graft.

D. Ossicles, cortical bone, cartilage or fascia (allograft/ xenograft)

Disadvantages	• Antigen reactions, therefore, rejection.
	• Transmission of infectious diseases

2. Synthetic Materials/Biomaterials

Synthetic materials are divided into two types.

A. Metals: Stainless steel, tantalum, platinum, titanium, and gold.

B. Non-metals: Subdivided into two groups:

     a. Plastics: 1. Solids, e.g. polyethylene, polytetrafluoroethylene (teflon), polydimethylsiloxane (silastic).

                     2. Porous, e.g. polytetrafluoroethylene carbon fibre composite (Proplast 1), polytetrafluoroethylene aluminium oxide composite (Proplast 2), high density polyethylene (Plastipre), ultrahigh molecular weight polythene (Polycel).

     b. Ceramics: These are inorganic crystal materials produced at high temperature, e.g.

                     1. Bioinert—aluminium oxide ceramics

2. Bioactive—calcium silicate glass ceramics
3. Biodegradable/bioresorbable hydroxy-apatite— tricalcium phosphate ceramics.

Advantages and Disadvantages

A. Metals—used in the form of wires.

Advantage • With natural materials give stability

Disadvantages • Formation of retraction pockets.
• Extrusion.
• Higher cost.

B. Non-metals

a. Plastics—commonly used are polyethylene. Teflon and plastipore.

Polyethylene and Teflon

Advantages • Solid plastic with smooth surfaces.
• No long-term inflammatory reactions.

Disadvantage • High chances of extrusion.

Plastipore • It has been used in total ossicular replacement.
Prosthesis (TORP) and partial ossicular replacement prosthesis (PORP).

Advantages • Easily available.
• Easily shaped.
• Easy to position.
• Easy to sterilize.
• Does not adhere.
• Efficient sound conductor.

Disadvantages • Can get slipped in the middle ear.
• High foreign body reaction hence rate of extrusion.

b. Ceramics:

Advantages • They are biocompatible and bio-functional.
• Easy to place and manipulate.

Disadvantage • Very costly.

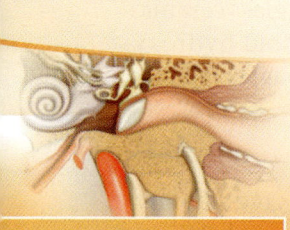

Innovative Cartilage Tympanoplasty

7

WHY CARTILAGE IS INNOVATIVE?

1. Availablity at operative site.
2. Stiffer consistency and easy to mould.
3. Minimum shrinkage and lateralization.
4. Natural angle of perichondrium for annular reconstruction.
5. Being mesenchymal lacks secreting glands and hair follicles, thus good for inlay graft.
6. Excellent elasticity and tension and has low metabolic rate.
7. Maintains volumetric integrity.
8. Minimum extrusion and absorbtion rate (1.19%).
9. Excellent graft takes up (96%).
10. Immune competent
11. No risk of HIV infection.
12. Inert and non-toxic.
13. Does not induce FB reactions.
14. Very cost-effective as compared to other synthetic grafts.
15. This is very effective material for TM reconstruction, ossicular reconstruction, osseous reconstruction and specially indicated in advanced middle ear pathology of atelectic, cholesteatoma and retraction pockets. It has a special role in reinforcement of TM in PORP and TORP procedures.

ADVANTAGES OF CARTILAGE IN OSSICULAR RECONSTRUCTION

1. Supports perichondrium and maintains aeration path to mastoid and round window.
2. No extrusion.
3. No lateralization.
4. No bony ankylosis.
5. No footplate subluxation.
6. Pressure contact is maintained.
7. No displacement
8. It separates perichondrium from silastic, hence less risk of silastic extrusion.
9. It has zero cost.
10. Accepted universally as a graft material.

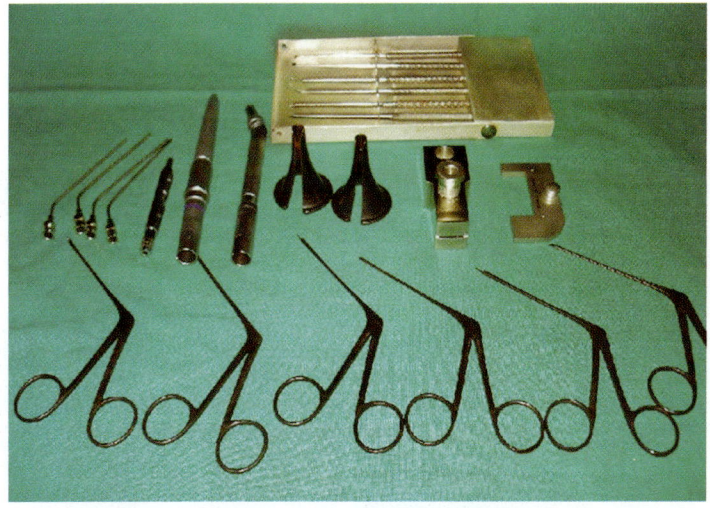

Fig. 7.1. Microsurgical instruments in cartilage tympanoplasty

TECHNIQUE OF HARVESTING TRAGAL CARTILAGE GRAFT

We present a modified harvesting approach for tragal perichondrium, used in tympanic membrane reconstruction. The technique described avoids amputation of the tragus thereby facilitating dissection of the perichondrium from the cartilage as compared to the traditional method. The approach described is technically easier, and removes any potential for cosmetic deformity associated with tragal cartilage amputation and reimplantation. Furthermore, both the anterior tragal perichondrium and the temporalis fascia remain intact, if further surgery is required. We recommend this approach for permeatal, tragal perichondrial grafting of small to medium sized tympanic membrane perforations.

SURGICAL PROCEDURE

The 1.5 cm incision is made 2 mm medially from the tragal crest line, so the scar will be hidden. The incision extends along the whole crest of the tragus from the helix to the antitragus. The skin is undermined and the tragus is dissected on both its sides as close as possible to the perichondrium. Tragal cresent must be maintained to avoid the tragal deformity (Fig. 7.2).

The whole tragus or only a part of it can be removed by cutting through the areolar tissue and cartilage. The cartilage should not be cut or crushed by scissor but cut with 11 or

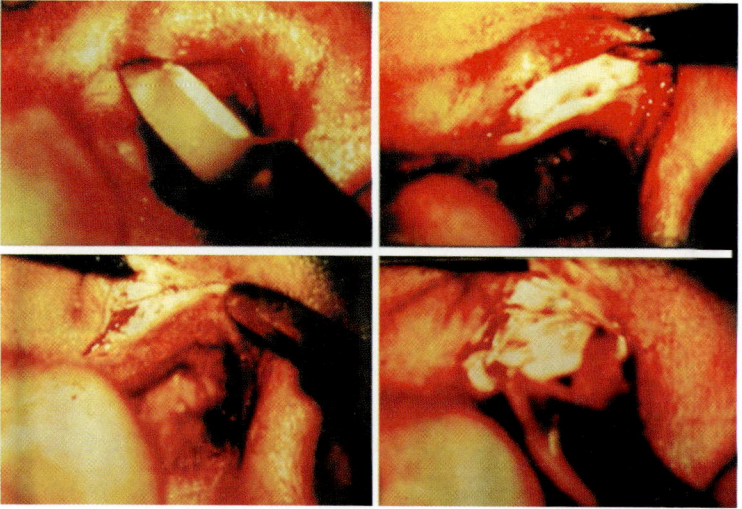

Fig. 7.2. Step-by-step surgical dissection for tragal cartilage perichondrium

15 No. knife. This will prevent the jeoparadising the peri-chondrium. The wound is closed with 3-onylon interrupted stitches. When the part of cartilage is used rest of the cartilage can be returned to the tragal site and will not give any tragal deformity. The dissected tragal cartilage and perichondrium is kept in saline until it is being used for reconstruction. The perichondrium can be elevated with Rosen circular knife. The cartilage with its perichondrium can be shaped according to the reconstruction planned.

SHAPING THE CARTILAGE STRUTS USING CARTILAGE SLICER

After harvesting the tragal cartilage, it is given different shapes and struts are prepared for required interpositioning in various tympanic and ossicular reconstructions. Using cartilage slicer (Fig. 7.3A) one can take the thinner slices which can be moulded during reconstruction (Figs 7.3B and 7.3C).

Following shapes are given to the cartilage in missing ossicles:

1. Small strut for necrosed lenticular process and stapes head.
2. L-shaped columella.
3. T-shaped columella.
4. Bow-shaped columella.
5. Boomrang columella. For ossicular assembly.
6. Y-shaped strut for malleus-footplate assembly.
7. Cartilage plates.

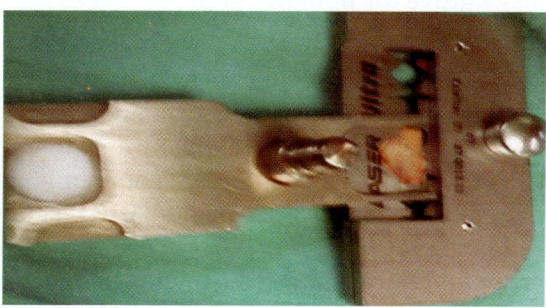

Fig. 7.3A. Cartilage slicer

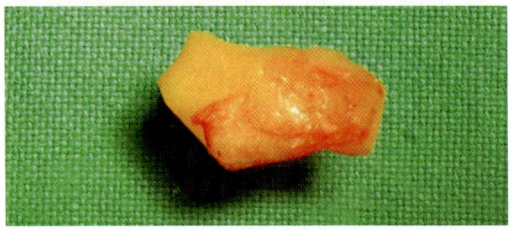

Fig. 7.3B. Sliced cartilage with perichondrium

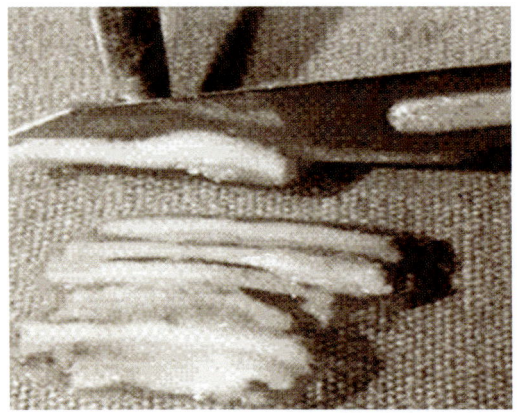

Fig. 7.3C. Cartilage strips with perichondrium

8. Vertical strips for palisade assembly
9. V-notch cartilage for shield graft.
10. Cartilage grove for Butterfly graft.

Preoperative Work-Up

The aim of the treatment must be to render a discharging ear dry, by conservative medical treatment and then perform middle ear reconstruction as per disease entity (myringoplasty or tympanoplasty). The ideal tympanoplasty restores sound protection for the round window by reconstructing a closed, air-containing middle ear against the round window membrane and restores sound pressure transformation for the oval window by connecting a large tympanic membrane or substitute membrane with stapes footplate via either an intact or reconstructed ossicular chain.

The detail ENT examination with otomicroscopy and suction clearance to be done preoperatively in each and every case. Medical treatment consists of broad-spectrum antibiotics, antihistaminics and anti-inflammatory drugs along with local antifungal and antibiotic-steroidal eardrops to be prescribed for 4 to 6 weeks prior to planned surgery.

Routine X-rays mastoid, CT scan, audiometry and bio-chemistry tests and wet gelfoam patch test as preoperative parameters should be done.

Septic foci in tonsils, adenoid and sinuses must be adequately treated for full two weeks before surgical intervention.

Xylocaine sensitivity test must be performed before surgery.

Gelfoam Patch Test

A gelfoam patch test (Fig. 7.4) is extremely useful before operative procedure. The preoperative audiogram is done and second audiogram is repeated after closing the perforation with a moist gelfoam. If the ossicular chain is intact and mobile, the hearing will improve.

The patch test also decides good hearing prediction, which site first to be done.

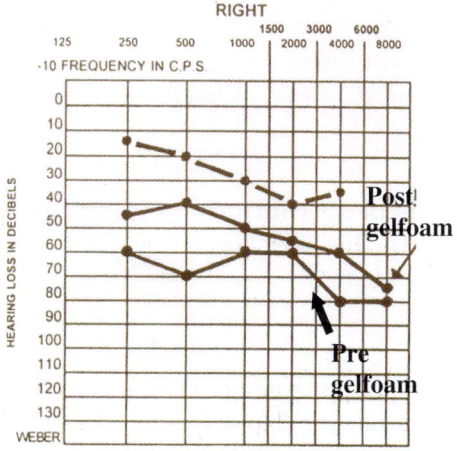

Fig. 7.4. Gelfoam patch test

INDICATIONS OF CARTILAGE TYMPANOPLASTY

In 2003, Bernal-Sprekelsen and co-workers recommended the following indications for cartilage tympanoplasty:

1. Total and subtotal perforations
2. Perforations with tympanosclerotic plaques
3. Perforation with atrophic membranes
4. Revision surgery for failed myringoplasty or tympanoplasty
5. Anterior and inferior perforation with tubal discharge
6. Retraction pockets
7. Partially or completely atelectatic tympanic membranes
8. Tympanic adherences
9. Revision surgery for failed tympanoplasty of type II and type III as well as tympanomastoidectomies

MIRKO TOS: CLASSIFICATIONS AND METHODS

Mirko Tos described 23 known cartilage tympanoplasty methods to reconstruct the eardrum and proposed a classification into six main groups. Following is the brief description of each method.

Group A

Cartilage tympanoplasty using palisades, strips, and slices. The eardrum is reconstructed by several, various, full-thickness pieces of cartilage with attached perichondrium on the ear canal side. In this group, six different methods are described.

Group B

Cartilage tympanoplasty with foils, thin plates, and thick plates, not covered with the perichondrium. In this group, four methods are included.

Group C

Tympanoplasty with cartilage-perichondrium composite island grafts. The perichondrium flap suspends or fixates the cartilage. In this group, four methods are included.

Group D

Tympanoplasty with special total pars tensa cartilage-perichondrium composite grafts. All three methods are used to close a total perforation, but differ from each. Three special methods are included in this group.

Group E

Cartilage-perichondrium composite island grafts tympanoplasty for anterior, inferior, and subtotal perforations. Two onlay and two underlay methods are included.

Group F

Special cartilage tympanoplasty methods: The cartilage disc is placed under the perforation—the perichondrium on to the denuded eardrum remnant.

POPULAR TECHNIQUES OF CARTILAGE TYMPANOPLASTY

Mainly four groups of cartilage tympanoplasty have been proposed in the literature by Mirko Tos. The choice of technique is determined by the surgeon's preference, size of the perforation, integrity of the ossicular chain, and the presence of cholesteatoma. The following techniques are commonly described in cartilage tympanoplasty.

1. Inlay butterfly technique.
2. Perichondrium-cartilage composite island technique
3. Perichondrium-cartilage shield technique.
4. Palisade technique

Comparison of Cartilage Graft with Other Grafts

There are few studies done on the cartilage graft tympanoplasty and its comparison with other materials as a control. The major studies which are close to our study are as follows: In 1997, John Dornhoffer performed 22 cartilage graft tympanoplasties and he observed that there was no residual perforation in this group. Control group was fascia/perichondrium graft (20 cases). He observed that there were residual perforations in 3 (15%) fascia/perichondrium tympanoplasties. Both series of patients had undergone type I tympanoplasty, and the middle ear pathology was considered to be similar between the two groups. The number of cases was too small for a case-control study.

Gerber studied 11 cartilage and 11 temporal fascia graft tympanoplasties in 2000 cases and observed comparable hearing results in both groups.

In 2004, Anderson performed 32 cartilage and 32 temporalis fascia graft tympanoplasties. He observed a 6% TM retraction in the cartilage group and a 36% TM retraction in the temporalis fascia group.

In 2004, Gierek performed 112 cases with cartilage and 30 cases with temporalis fascia. He observed that there was no significant hearing difference between the two groups.

In 2005, Couloinger, observed 59 cartilage graft tympanoplasties and 20 temporalis fascia graft tympanoplasties and reported no postoperative hearing difference between the two groups.

Tympanoplasty is a common surgical procedure for treatment of chronic otitis media. Although the temporalis fascia is considered the best grafting material, various surgeons have used alternatives to simplify the grafting procedure. In general, cartilage graft is the most predictable material of choice for ear surgeries and can be used as an alternative to fascia graft.

CARTILAGE TYMPANOPLASTY—OPERATIVE PROCEDURES

In this monograph, mainly four techniques have been described for cartilage tympanoplasty, namely the inlay butterfly graft, perichondrium/cartilage composite island graft, palisade graft, and cartilage shield graft.

Surgical Approaches

1. Post-aural
2. End-aural
3. Endomeatal
4. Transcanal transtympanic
5. Canalplasty in narrow EAC

Methods and Techniques

1. Inlay Butterfly Graft Technique

Eavey(1998) described an original technique that involves placing a specially shaped cartilage-perichondrium composite graft both under and on to the eardrum. Thus this technique is partly inlay and partly onlay. However, most of the graft is on the level of perforation as an inlay graft and the technique is called inlay. The circumferentially incised edges of the cartilage curl apart, like wings of a butterfly and hence the name "inlay butterfly technique".

Indications

Small- or medium-sized dry perforations with an intact ossicular chain: For closure of a non-marginal tympanic membrane perforation, currently popular techniques utilize either an underlay or an onlay approach. However, both procedures require incising canal skin. A transcanal inlay procedure could provide theoretical advantages of ease, speed, and comfort. Specifically designed cartilage that will facilitate the transcanal approach similar to placement of a solid tube is employed and evaluated. A transcanal cartilage butterfly inlay technique is found to be efficient and effective to close a subgroup of small-to-medium-sized tympanic membrane perforations including cases in which the condition of the tympanic membrane is somewhat hostile. Postoperative patient comfort is an additional benefit. The technique is faster and less expensive. No external ear canal packing or support for the graft in the tympanic cavity is required because the graft is instantly stable. The procedure is minimally invasive.

Patient Selection and Preoperative Preparation (Fig. 7.5)

The patient with age of >13 years, both gender, and chronic otitis media (mucosal-inactive) with central perforation of >50% and those requiring revision surgeries for failed myringoplasty are included for surgery.

The patient is given oral ciprofloxacin 500 milligram 12 hourly one day prior surgery and continued till 10th

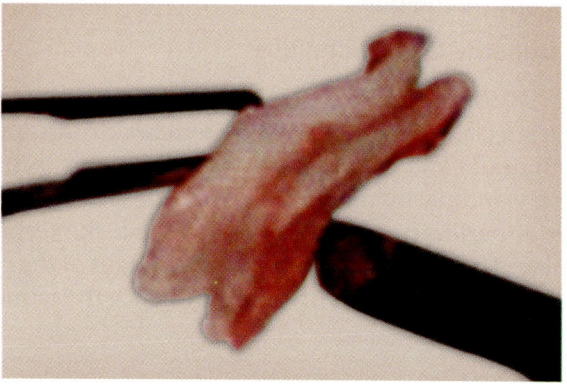

Fig. 7.5. Preparation of butterfly graft in cartilageplasty

postoperative day. Since the surgery is performed under local anaesthesia, so the patient is sedated with pethidine and promethazine intramuscularly as per body weight.

Surgical Technique

The patient is given 5–10 ml of 2% xylocaine with 1:1,00,000 adrenaline injection as per the approach selected, for four quadrant canal wall and tragus is infiltrated. About 2 cm vertical incision is given by number 15 scalpel from incisura terminalis up to intratragal notch which is around 5 mm medial to the tip of the tragus. The single stroke skin incision is given up to tragus cartilage. The assistant holds the tissue of the tip of the tragus by non-toothed forceps or skin hooks and clears the surgical field from blood by suction. Whereas the operating surgeon holds the skin with non-toothed forceps or skin hooks and then the cartilage along with perichondrium is dissected with cartilage scissors. Similarly, cartilage along with perichondrium from the anterior aspect of tragal cartilage is dissected and thus made free at incisura terminalis.

The cartilage along with the perichondrium is excised with number 15 scalpel giving incision from incisura terminalis once the cartilage size of 2 cm in length and 1.5 cm in breadth is obtained. Thus, the cartilage is harvested. The skin is closed with 4/0 prolene interrupted suture. Then, the graft is kept on silastic block. The perichondrium away from canal is elevated with number 15 scalpel and removed. For creating the butterfly, number 11 scalpel is used and thus created around 1.5 mm groove along the circumferential border of the cartilage disc allowing the cartilage flanges to spring open. If the handle of malleus and/or the incudostapedial joint is visible then we remove the V-shaped cartilage partly to allow place for handle of malleus and incudo-stapedial joint.

After the perforation rim is freshened, the cartilage graft can then be anchored on to the perforation similar to a tympanostomy tube (Fig. 7.6). A split thickness skin graft can be placed over the graft, if the perforation is large. Cartilage butterfly graft inlay tympanoplasty is effective in the vast majority of patients with moderate to large perforations.

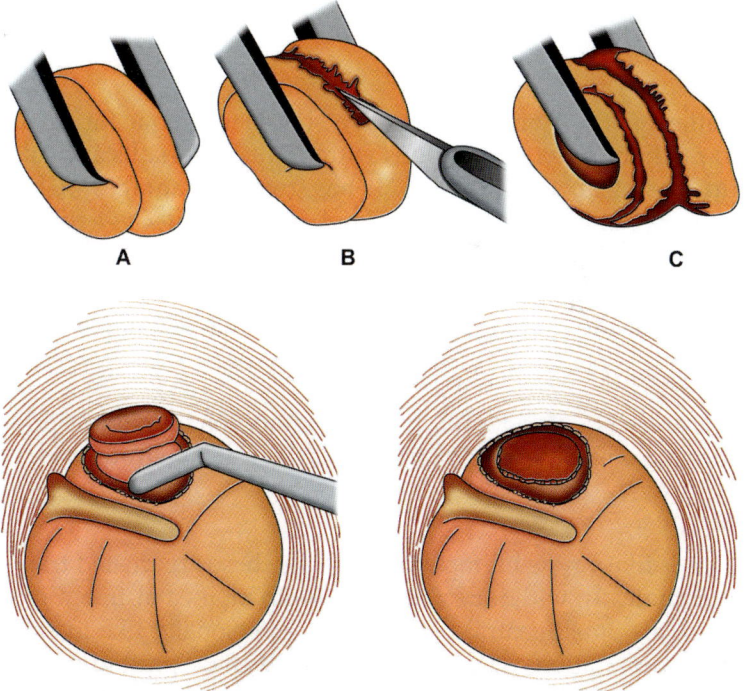

Fig. 7.6. Placement of butterfly graft in perforation

Postoperative Care and Follow-Up

The patient is prescribed tab ciprofloxacin 500 mg 12 hourly for 10 days. The ribbon gauge pack and the stitch is removed on 7th postoperative day. The remaining gelatin sponge is suctioned on the same 7th postoperative day. Then, the patient is prescribed chloramphenicol and dexamethasone eardrops for six weeks. The patient is again followed up after 2 weeks, 6 weeks and 12 weeks. The hearing is assessed on 12 weeks.

Audiological Evaluation

For the hearing assessment, pure tone audiogram is done seven days prior to operation and then 12 weeks after the operation. The audiological results are reported according to American Academy of Otolaryngology—Head and Neck Surgery guidelines.

Results of Butterfly Graft Tympanoplasty

Butterfly inlay tympanoplasty is a simple technique for small-to-medium-sized perforations with gratifying results and take up rate of up to 92 to 96%. It has great advantages of less operative time, day care surgery and can be accepted as a routine procedure in day-to-day practice.

2. Composite Cartilage Perichondrium Graft Technique

Indications

The anterior, inferior and subtotal perforations, residual perforation, non-healing perforations and high-risk perforations.

Surgical Technique

This is like a type I tympanoplasty. All these are treated trans-tympanically without raising the tympanomeatal flap. Since these are small central perforations, I personally like to close these perforations by using composite cartilage graft technique (Fig. 7.7A). The middle ear is filled with gelfoam and harvested composite graft is placed through the perforation and spread as inlay graft. The perichondrium will remain under the remnant of incised edges of tympanic perforation. The graft is covered with antibiotic soaked gelfoam balls. The silastic sheet is placed over the new graft as a support. In large central, subtotal or total perforations, I always like to use large tympanomeatal flap for composite cartilage tympanoplasty (Fig. 7.7B). The ossicular integrity is always tested before the placement of the graft. The graft take is 95 to 96% with excellent hearing. The use of angle endoscope is an additional asset to look into minute pathology which may be hidden.

In ears with advanced pathology, the functional and anatomical results of surgery are compromised by such factors

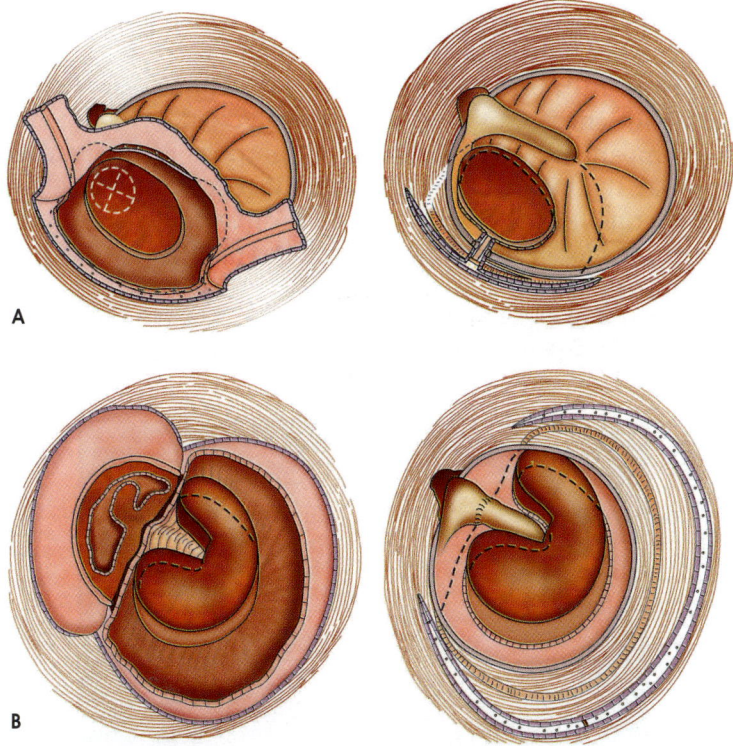

Fig. 7.7. (A) Perichondrium cartilage composite island graft in small perforation
(B) Perichondrium cartilage composite graft in central perforation

as total perforation, tympanosclerosis, atelectasis, suppuration, or previous surgery. Perichondrium cartilage composite grafts (PCCGs) were used for membrane grafting in 600 cases. The graft was obtained from the tragus and/or the concha.

Closure of the eardrum perforation was successful in 96% of the procedures. An air-bone gap of less than or equal to 30 dB was obtained in 92.4% of tympanoplasty type I procedures and in 87% of tympanoplasty type III procedures. The conclusion drawn from the results is that PCCG is a reliable graft in cases of advanced destruction of the middle ear.

The author presents his experience with large cartilage-perichondrial composite grafts used to reconstruct total tympanic membrane perforations in 150 ears. Patients chosen for this procedure had failed earlier tympanoplasty surgery or were identified as poor candidates for conventional fascia tympanoplasty because of the perforation size.

Successful perforation closure was achieved in 96% of ears with chronic otitis media characterized by absence of the tympanic membrane, including portions of the anterior annular ligament. Hearing results in general were good, considering the advanced stage of the disease, which required the use of alloplastic ossicular prostheses (PORP and TORP) in 76% of ears.

The present experience with conchal cartilage tympanoplasty demonstrates that the procedure is very effective, particularly

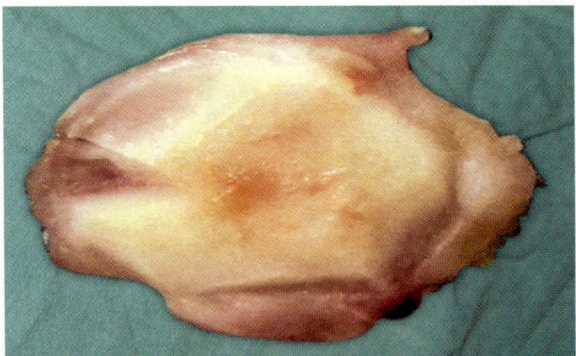

Fig. 7.8. Composite conchal cartilage graft tympanoplasty—conchal island graft

in total perforations, atelectasis, isolated tympanic membrane perforations, and wet perforation drainage during surgery. The conchal cartilage underlay graft resulted in a 95% take rate and no lateralization or displacement in middle ear. The follow-up period was three years.

Although the graft-take success rate is high in cartilage tympanoplasty, hearing gain might not be satisfactory due to its effect on tympanic membrane elasticity. However, despite the belief of many surgeons, recent studies have shown that no statistically significant difference exists in temporalis fascia and cartilage tympanoplasties in terms of postoperative hearing results. In conclusion, the conchal cartilage island graft tympanoplasty is an effective procedure for all types of tympanoplasty procedure. It provides better graft take and hearing results, if it is properly prepared and placed (Fig. 7.9).

Results of Composite Cartilage Graft Tympanoplasty

Hearing improvement was maximal at 2000 Hz regardless of the method of ossicular reconstruction. Closure of the air-bone gap at this frequency to within 10 dB was achieved in 82% of type I tympanoplasty, 72% of type III tympanoplasty (PORP), and 70% of type III (TORP) tympanoplasty. Although cartilage

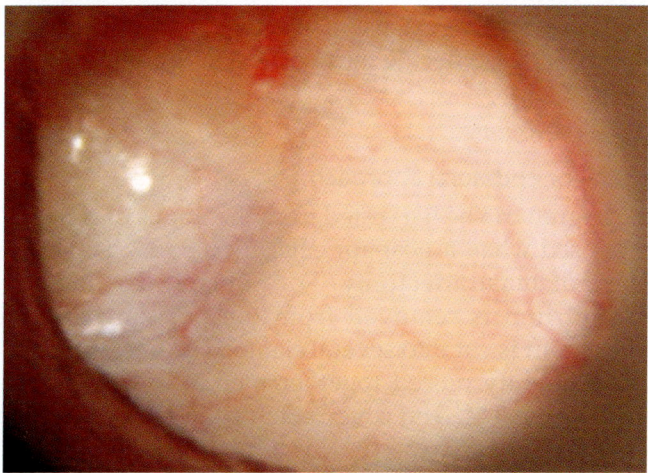

Fig. 7.9. Final appearance of conchal composite cartilage graft after 12 weeks

autografts have also been promoted to reverse tympanic membrane atelectasis, the authors believe that the above preoperative conditions are strong indications for this grafting technique.

3. Palisade Technique with Cartilage and Perichondrium and Composite Graft

Indications

Recurrent tympanic membrane perforations are usually caused by underlying conditions such as an adhesive process with a poorly aerated middle ear space, a thermal perforation, infection, or technical error at the time of graft placement. Despite surgical treatment, these reperforations pose a significant otologic problem that may lead to the development of chronic otitis media and cholesteatoma. The purpose of this study is to detail the use of a new cartilage palisade tympanoplasty technique that has yielded a 100% tympanic membrane closure rate without recurrent perforations. The acoustic properties of the rebuilt tympanic membrane were analyzed for types I, II, and III tympanoplasty and revealed a significant improvement in the postoperative air–bone gap. The surgical techniques are adapted to location and size of perforation as well as extension of active disease. The ossicular pathology will also decide the choice of surgical technique.

Surgical Technique

Post-aural or end-aural approach

Cartilage graft can be harvested from the tragus or concha. The latter is used when a post-auricular incision is planned, as in the case of mastoidectomy. For conchal cartilage graft, perichondrium is removed from the post-auricular side. Cartilage graft is cut into several slanted slices or strips, which are subsequently pieced together medial to the malleus to reconstruct the TM. The covex side of the palisade is turned towards the tympanic cavity. This technique is favoured when ossicular chain reconstruction is performed because it provides a better visualization of the prosthesis and precise placement of graft on to the prosthesis. In cases of posterior perforation, the anterior half of the TM can be left alone to allow post-operative surveillance and future myringotomy tube placement.

The palisade cartilage technique is suitable to manage difficult pathologic conditions in middle ear surgery. It was demons-trated that the palisade cartilage technique can be combined safely with titanium ossicular replacement prostheses. Regarding postoperative hearing results, the negative preselection of pathologic conditions must be considered.

Underlay palisade for large perforation

In this technique, the tympanomeatal flap is raised in posterior perforation. The edge of the perforation with the keratinized epithelium is excised. The skin incision is placed relatively laterally in the ear canal. A large tympanomeatal flap is elevated together with the fibrous annulus and the remnants of the posterior half of eardrum and the epithelium covering the posterior half of the malleus handle. The palisades are placed on to the inferoposterior bony annulus. The first palisade is placed on the posterior edge of the malleus handle, superiorly. All the palisades are placed close, but not on to the bony annulus. The results are excellent in closure of perforation.

Only palisade for total and subtotal perforation

Indications for onlay palisade technique are the same as underlay technique. There are reperforations, cholesteatoma in adults and children, retraction pockets, adhesive otitis media, thick and secretory middle ear mucosa, ear with poor tubal functions.

In total or subtotal perforations, there are three onlay techniques wherein cartilage palisades can be used, as (1) onlay technique with elevation of three superior epithelial flaps, (2) onlay technique with elevation of large tympanomeatal skin flap and epithelial flaps, (3) Technique with outward elevation of the epithelium and the skin flap. All the palisades are placed close, but not on to the bony annulus. The long-term efficacy of cartilage palisades in the reconstruction of posterosuperior retraction pockets has been well documented in clinical studies. The results of this onlay technique are extremely satisfactory

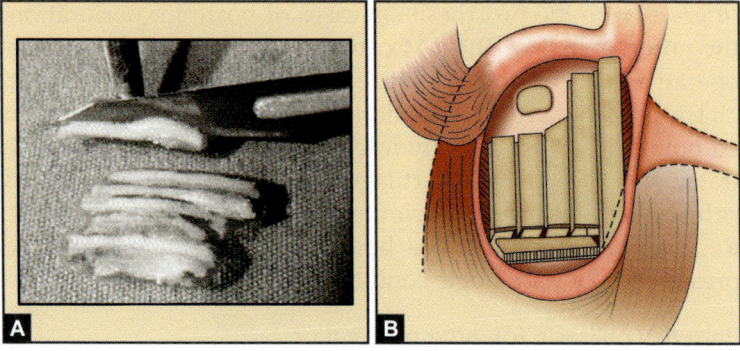

Fig. 7.10. Palisade technique in different perforations: (A) Slanted palisades; (B) Horizontal palisades

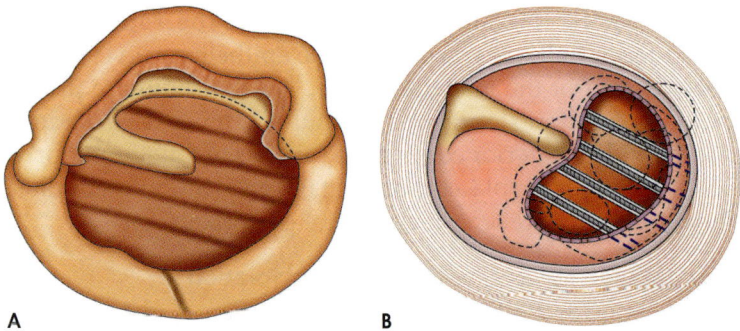

A

B

Fig. 7.11. Vertical palisades for central and total perforations: (A) Total perforation; (B) Central perforation

both anatomical and auditory gain point of view. All types of anterior, inferior, subtotal and total perforations can be closed with excellent results (Figs 7.10 and 7.11).

Results of Palisade Tympanoplasty

The graft take rate was 100%. There were no extrusions of prostheses. The palisade cartilage technique is suitable to manage difficult pathologic conditions in middle ear surgery. It was demonstrated that the palisade cartilage technique can be combined safely with titanium ossicular replacement prostheses. Regarding postoperative hearing results, the negative preselection of pathologic conditions must be considered. The comparison of fascia and cartilage palisade grafting for drum reconstruction after tensa cholesteatoma surgery in children indicates that the palisade technique may be superior in respect to prevention of drum retraction and perforation. Further, in sinus cholesteatoma surgery, the long-term hearing results are better when grafting with cartilage palisades.

4. Cartilage Shield Graft Technique

Surgical Technique

Post-aural or end-aural approach

Cartilage shield tympanoplasty is a procedure for repairing total tympanic membrane perforations. This procedure is indicated primarily for patients with total perforations, severely atelectatic tympanic membranes, and failures of previous tympanoplasty associated with chronic eustachian tube dysfunction. Although the graft take of this technique has been reported to be excellent, there have been concerns regarding hearing results because it replaces the entire tympanic membrane with cartilage. A vascular strip incision is made in the ear canal, followed by a post-auricular incision. Areolar tissue overlying temporal fascia is harvested. A round piece of conchal cartilage is harvested and perichondrium on both sides is removed. A small wedge of cartilage is removed to accommodate the handle of the malleus. The graft is then placed medial to the malleus and the remnants of the tympanic membrane. The areolar graft is then placed in between the cartilage graft and the remnant of tympanic membrane (Figs 7.12 and 7.13).

Graft take was achieved (100%). No statistically significant association between the postoperative pure tone average–air bone gap results and age, sex, or type of tympanoplasty was observed (p>0.05). The overall mean preoperative pure tone average – air bone gap was 27.0 ±10.5 dB, and it decreased to 14.9 ± 7.0 dB 3 months postoperatively. A statistically significant improvement was observed. Excellent graft take results were

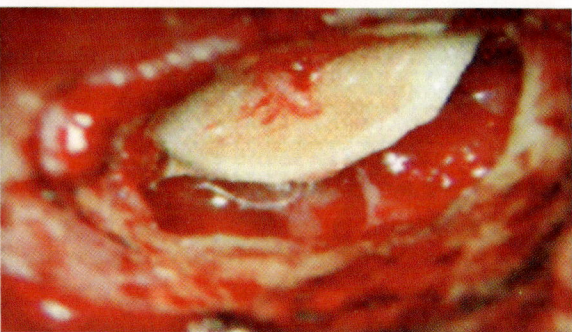

Fig. 7.12. Composite cartilage shield graft

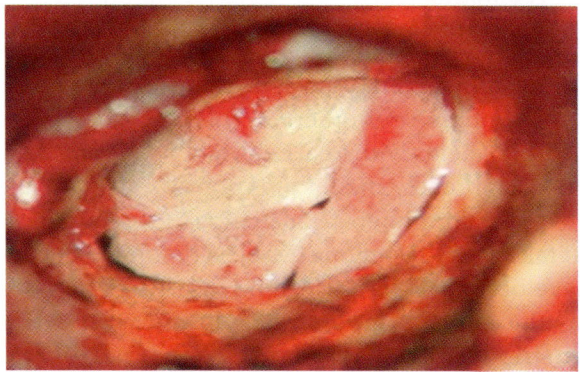

Fig. 7.13. Composite cartilage graft with thick plates

achieved and hearing outcomes were satisfactory. Therefore, shield cartilage graft is a valid alternative in all tympanoplasty procedures.

CARTILAGE SHIELD T-TUBE GRAFT (Fig. 7.14)

Indication for Cartilage Shield T-Tube Tympanoplasty

The main indication is in chronic Eustachian tube dysfunction.

Procedure

This technique is described by Prof. JL Dornhoffer in 1999. In this technique, the cartilage is harvested from the tragus and used in total pars tensa defect. The cartilage perichondrium composite graft is divided into posteriot and anterior island. The cartilage is surrounded by a belt of perichondrium. In the anterior island graft, a hole is made in the cartilage for T-tube using a round knife. Then with straight pick, the hole is enlarged for T-tube placement. The T-tube is remodelled by trimming the flanges to 3 to 4 mm. Finally, the T-tube is placed in the cartilage window and brought out through the perichondrial

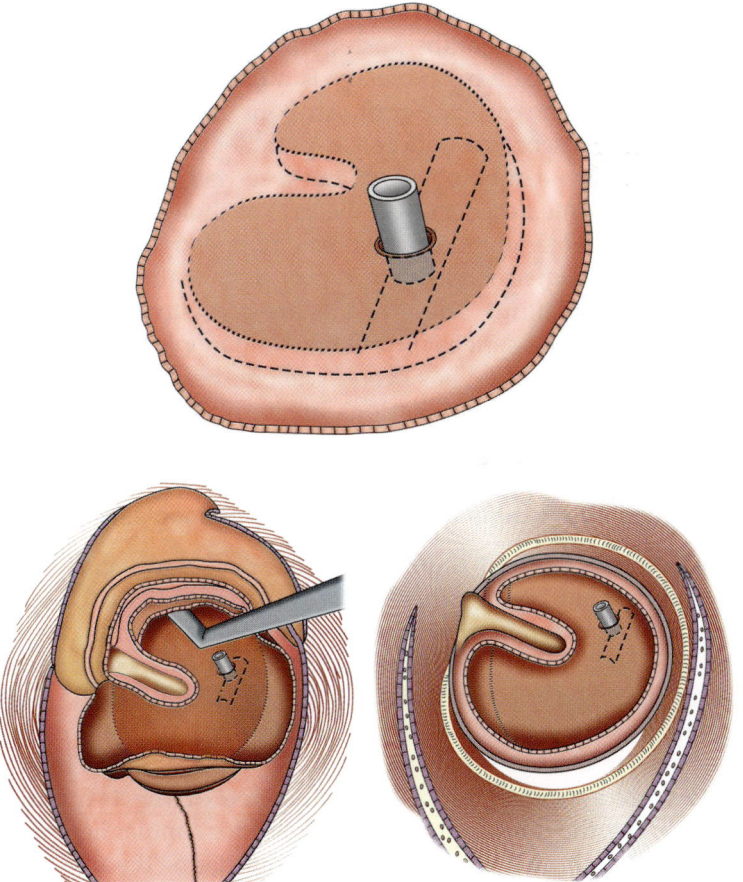

Fig. 7.14. The cartilage shield T-tube tympanoplasty

surface. The graft is now ready to be placed into the tympanic cavity. The patients with T-tube needs long-term follow-up after surgery. By this technique, the chronic eustachian tube function can be corrected with excellent results.

Postoperative Care

Antibiotics and anti-inflammatory drugs along with steriod are prescribed for two weeks. Topical antibiotic drops are initiated for 2 weeks after surgery. The canal wick is removed after one week and canal gelfoam is removed from the EAC. Audiogram is obtained in 3–4 months postoperative, mainly to evaluate air-bone gap since tympanometry is no longer reliable due to the rigidity of the cartilage graft. Air-bone gap is a good tool to assess the presence of middle ear pathology. If required, CT temporal bone can be obtained and a second look procedure can be performed especially in the case of cholesteatoma.

Our experience with cartilage shield tympanoplasty demons-trates a high degree of reliability, especially for patients at higher risk for graft failure. These results are consistent with other similar published series on cartilage tympanoplasty. The graft take of this technique has been excellent, hearing results are satisfactory, and complications are minimal. We strongly recommend this technique to our otological colleagues.

Postoperative Results in Shield Graft Tympanoplasty

The authors present their experience with large cartilage-perichondrial composite grafts used to reconstruct total tympanic membrane perforations in 300 ears. Patients chosen for this procedure had failed earlier tympanoplasty surgery or were identified as poor candidates for conventional fascia graft tympanoplasty because of the perforation size. Successful perforation closure was achieved in 97% of ears with chronic otitis media characterized by absence of the tympanic membrane, including portions of the anterior annular ligament. Hearing results in general were good, considering the advanced stage of the disease, which required the use of alloplastic ossicular prostheses (PORP and TORP) in 75% of ears. Hearing improvement was maximal at 2000 Hz regardless of the method of ossicular reconstruction. Closure of the air-bone gap at this frequency to within 10 dB was achieved in 85% of type I tympanoplasties, 75% of type III (PORP), and 70% of type III (TORP) tympanoplasties. Although cartilage autografts have also been promoted to reverse tympanic membrane atelectasis, the authors believe that the above preoperative conditions are strong indications for this grafting technique.

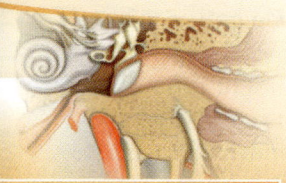

Current Concepts in Paediatric Cartilage Tympanoplasty

8

Tympanoplasty in children is a current and controversial theme. The success of tympanoplasty traditionally has been measured only by the postoperative integrity of the graft. Yet, there are other variables that may be used to determine success. The objectives of the present work is to analyze which factors are predictive of successful tympanoplasty in paediatric patients and to construct and validate a prognostic index that could be used as a tool to predict the success of tympanoplasty in children.

The first known attempt to repair an eardrum perforation was allegedly made by Banzer, in 1640, using a swine bladder membrane graft. In 1853, Toynbee introduced the "artificial eardrum", a small rubber disc with a silver rod—to facilitate introduction and extraction. In 1878, Berthold used a skin graft and in 1887, Blake recommended the use of a piece of paper as a template to tympanic membrane regeneration. Notwithstanding, it was only after 1944, with the beginning of antibiotics and with the improvement in surgical techniques that other materials were used as grafts in tympanoplasties. After this time, in 1952, Zollner and Wullstein published their methods, using retroauricular skin grafts; however, they did not succeed in treating tympanic membrane perforations.

The cartilage perichondrium composite graft (CPCG) was used to close the tympanic membrane perforation. Successful drum closure was achieved in 86.6% of cases, regardless of the site of perforation or the status of the operated ear. The graft was taken from the tragus and was placed in an underlay fashion with cartilage towards the promontory and the perichondrium immediately under the tympanic membrane remnants. The postoperative hearing gain although delayed up to 6 months was excellent either subjective or objective. So, CPCG has proved advantageous as a graft material to close perforation in the tympanic membrane in paediatric age group.

Paediatric tympanoplasty is a frequently performed procedure with varying reported success rates ranging between 65 and 85%. In general, tympanic membrane repair success in children is often perceived as lagging behind what is typically achieved in adults having similar underlying risk factors. Previously quoted reasons for the poorer success rate include: frequent upper respiratory tract infections, persistent otitis media and ongoing Eustachian tube dysfunction, and inconsistent postoperative care.

Graft choice in paediatric tympanoplasty (fascia versus cartilage) has not been examined to the extent that it has in the adult population where its use has been justified by excellent outcomes in numerous reports. In 2003, Dornhoffer published a retrospective review of 1000 adult and paediatric patients that underwent cartilage tympanoplasty for all indications wherein a high perforation closure rate (96%) was noted with significantly improved hearing. The earlier reports also revealed cartilage to be no different than with fascia with respect to hearing outcomes. Mohamad concluded that cartilage tympanoplasty was associated with significantly better rates of tympanic membrane repair while resulting in hearing outcomes that were no different. If one accepts these findings, the logical question follows as to why cartilage cannot reasonably be considered an acceptable default reconstruction material for most cases of tympanoplasty.

One possible source of hesitation in routinely using cartilage for paediatric tympanoplasty is the limited data available on the long-term outcomes and collective uncertainty regarding the appropriate timing of tympanoplasty relative to age. Among publications that have examined the significance of age as a prognostic value in paediatric tympanoplasty, the majority utilized fascia grafts for repair of the tympanic membrane and many lacked high numbers of paediatric patients. Thus, the purpose of this study is to explore long-term paediatric cartilage tympanoplasty outcomes with particular attention given to age. In doing so, we substantiate the hypothesis that, when patients are selected judiciously based on perceived underlying Eustachian tube maturity, outstanding hearing and perforation closure rates can be safely attained when cartilage is used as the standard default tympanoplasty grafting material in the paediatric population.

Decision about timing of tympanoplasty was undertaken according to the guidelines developed at our institution as tympanoplasty is not considered until patients are at least 10 years of age. If the contralateral middle ear is found to be abnormal, then adenotonsillectomy and nasal treatment are advised. But tympanoplasty is recommended only after age of 10 years, by then upper respiratory tract is well stabilized.

Thus, numerous types of tympanoplasty grafts have been described. The most commonly used techniques for graft placement on the tympanic membrane are the "underlay" (medial) and "onlay" (lateral), and the most used types of graft are the temporal muscle fascia and perichondrium, with similar success rates (approximately 90%). Among children, these rates vary between 66 and 93.5% with the use of temporal fascia graft. However, these two techniques require a skin incision in the external acoustic meatus (EAM), which causes greater morbidity and the need for better postoperative care, reducing the use of these techniques in children. In 1989, Gross described the "inlay" approach, with the use of a fat tissue plug for small perforations, however, without success in repairing the perforations.

The cartilage was first used to rebuild the ossicular chain in 1958 by Jansen. Some years later, this material started to be used as a graft in tympanoplasties, especially in cases of advanced middle ear diseases, because of their robustness, offering greater resistance to resorptions. In 1998, Eavey described tympanoplasty in children using the tragal cartilage and bilateral perichondrium (cartilage plug) and the placement of a graft without incisions in the EAM (inlay approach). This new approach, when compared to the previous ones, showed a number of advantages for its use in children: no need for a tympanic-meatal flap, reducing pain and the need for post-operative care; possibility of placing the graft in the so-called "hostile" eardrums (those with tympanosclerosis plaques and malleus exposure); shorter surgical time, it can be carried out under general anaesthesia without orotracheal intubation, thus giving the patient the possibility of an early hospital discharge—and reducing costs—no need to dress the EAM, since the graft fits stable on to the eardrum.

This study was conducted at KEM hospital by postaural or endoural approach using underlay cartilage technique. Specifically, if the perforation exceeded half of the tympanic membrane, a single large (6–7 mm diameter) **circular composite perichondrium-cartilage island graft** was utilized with perichondrium having been stripped off of the medial surface of the graft. If the perforation was small and limited to either the posterior or anterior portion of the tympanic membrane, either a single **semicircular composite perichondrium-cartilage island graft or a palisade** of small bare cartilage grafts subsequently covered with a piece of perichondrium was utilized. In few cases with small perforation, a **butterfly graft** was used with excellent results.

Management of tympanic membrane perforations in the paediatric population is a common challenge and optimization of surgical technique for repair of these perforations is an ever-emerging field. The tympanic membrane repair success rate in this study was quite high with an average of 80 to 85% with a mean follow-up of greater than 3 to 5 years. This result compared favourably even to most of what has been published on adult tympanoplasty, thereby reaffirming the practice of using cartilage as the default tympanic membrane graft repair material in lieu of fascia at the KEM Hospital Pune. As it is becoming more clear that the use of cartilage as a grafting material for tympanoplasty results in improved results while avoiding significant impairment in hearing outcomes as compared to fascia, cartilage tympanoplasty appears to be becoming more common in children. Possible benefits of cartilage grafts over fascia that may account for improved outcomes include a relative tendency to rigidly fixate and avoid medial migration during the postoperative healing phase as well as a tendency to resist re-retraction when underlying Eustachian tube dysfunction is pervasive.

Our observation revealed the use of butterfly cartilage inlay graft in patients with medium to large perforations was excellent achieving a success rate of 80% with most patients experiencing an improvement in hearing postoperatively. Despite our enthusiasm for cartilage tympanoplasty, which has become the most frequently used tympanic membrane repair material in our practice for both adults and children, its use is not without negative consequences. First, if care is not taken when harvesting the graft, a donor-site cosmetic deformity may result. This is particularly true with respect to the tragus where preserving a residual lateral crescent of cartilage (ideally at least 2 mm) is recommended. Second, assessment of the middle ear status by tympanometry is not useful following cartilage tympanoplasty due to the effects of its stiffness on tympanic membrane compliance. Third, opaque cartilage grafts render otoscopic view of the middle ear cleft impossible.

Lastly, tympanic membrane intubation may be difficult following cartilage tympanoplasty. In our experience, a laser may be helpful in executing a myringotomy when tube placement is required. All of these potential negative consequences notwithstanding, it is our impression that the upside of cartilage grafts is sufficient to justify their routine use in children. A prospective controlled study would be required to definitively establish this point. The audiometric configuration revealed excellent ABG closure in routinely performed cartilage tympanoplasty.

DISCUSSION

Cartilage, as well as fascia, vein and periosteum are mesenchymal tissues and, for this very reason, they do not scale off. They have no secretory glands, nor hair follicles as those found in the skin, thus being used as tympanic membrane graft without the risk of causing iatrogenic cholesteatomas.

Contrary to other materials, cartilage has some physical properties that facilitate its use in tympanoplasties. These grafts are nourished by diffusion and easily incorporated on the tympanic membrane, which has been confirmed in second look tympanoplasties. It is a more robust material, easier to fit on the eardrum perforation site. It is thicker, less prone to resorption and retraction. Nonetheless, the cartilage acoustic transfer characteristics are theoretically worse because of its thickness. In 2000, Zahnert et al. carried out an experimental study concluding that a 500 μm thick cartilage has an acceptable acoustic transfer capacity with good mechanical stability.

Success rates of tympanic membrane perforation closure with cartilage plugs in adults are high. In 2000, Testa et al. published a closure success rate of 96.8% with hearing improvement in all the cases. Lubianca-Neto et al., in 2000, published rates of 90% and 94.4%, respectively. These are the goals to be reached in children.

Notwithstanding, low immunity, high upper airway infection rate and Eustachian tube dysfunction are factors responsible for reducing the success rates of tympanoplasties in the paediatric population.

CONCLUSIONS

In conclusion, we note that the use of cartilage in paediatric type I tympanoplasty for tympanic membrane perforation repair results in excellent outcomes that are comparable to the best-case outcomes that have been reported in the adult population. Furthermore, it appears that when paediatric cartilage tympanoplasty is timed according to perceived underlying Eustachian tube maturity, age does not impact the rate of tympanic membrane repair or hearing outcomes. The proposed study provides the paediatrician and the otolaryngologist a tool with which to quantify the probability of success that a patient, who presents with chronic perforation of the tympanic membrane and requires surgical intervention.

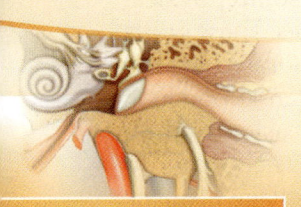

Clinical Applications in Cartilage Tympanoplasty
(KEM-Study) (1980 to 2010)

9

The study design consists of 600 cases of varied middle ear pathologies of safe and unsafe type. In our study, 450 cases were primary and 150 cases were revision surgery. The age group was 10 to 65 and males were 54% and females were 46%. Majority cases were done under LA (480) and rest under GA (120). All paediatric cases were done under GA (Tables 9.1 and 9.2).

Table 9.1. Surgical approaches

Sr. no	Approaches	Cases	%
1.	End-aural	312	52
2.	Endomeatal	192	32
3.	Post-aural	60	10
4.	Transtymp	36	06
	Total	**600**	**100**

Table 9.2. Anaesthesia: Gen/Local + Sedation

Sr. no.	Anaesthesia	Cases	%
1.	General	120	20
2.	Local	480	80
	Total	**600**	**100**

Routine preoperative work-up was done which includes haemogram urine, biochemical tests, serology X-ray mastoid, X-ray PNS and preoperative audiograms. The medical and anaesthesia fitness was sought before surgery.

TECHNIQUE OF LOCAL ANAESTHESIA

1. The concha is pulled anteriorly and 0.5 ml of 2% xylocaine with adrenaline (1;200000) is injected in the post-auricular fold.
2. The same needle is introduced subcutaneously under the posterior ear canal skin and 0.5 ml local anaesthetic is injected.
3. The same needle is introduced through the same original point in the inferior direction towards inferior wall of the ear canal and 0.5 ml local anaesthetic is injected.
4. The same needle is introduced towards the superior wall of the ear canal and 0.5 ml local anaesthetic is injected.
5. The external meatus is opened by small killian speculum and 0.5 ml is injected at 12, 3, 6 and 9 o'clock positions.
6. The middle ear mucosa is anaesthetised with 10% local spray or 4% xylocaine with adrenaline-soaked gelfoam.

Techniques in Tympanic Reconstruction

1. Onlay technique.
2. Inlay technique.

Onlay Technique

The sliced perichondrium cartilage is placed on outer surface of the denuded drum remnant.

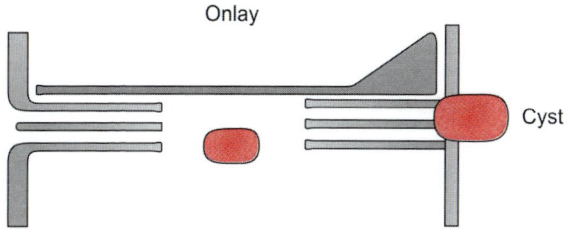

Onlay

Cyst

Disadvantages
1. Blunting.
2. Lateralization.
3. Epithelial cyst formation.

Inlay Technique

The sliced perichondriun is placed underneath the drum remnant. This is most common technique in use world over.

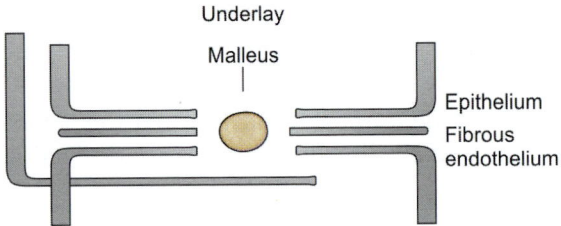

Advantages
1. No blunting.
2. No lateralization.
3. No burying of epithelium

Disadvantages
1. Residual perforation (anterior, subtotal and total)
2. Medialization.
3. Chronic myringitis.
4. Tympanosclerosis

STUDY DESIGN AND STUDY GROUPS
(600 CASES)

1. Myringoplasty   (300)
2. Ossiculoplasty   (110)
3. Ossiousplasty (bony defect)   (70)
4. Mastoid obliteration   (120)

1. MYRINGOPLASTY (300 CASES)

Transcanal–Transtympanic Approach

Surgical Technique

Cartilage tympanoplasty was performed by the senior author in a manner similar to the techniques described in the literature. Either a transcanal or postauricular approach is used to access the tympanic membrane and middle ear. After the tympanic membrane pathology has been assessed, the tragus is injected with a local anaesthetic. An incision along the free edge of the tragus is performed and the subcutaneous tissue is dissected to the lateral border of the cartilage and its perichondrium. The cartilage is then widely exposed on both its lateral and medial surfaces and then harvested with its attached perichondrium; the donor site is then closed. Conchal cartilage has been used less frequently, but is harvested with ease through an anterior or posterior approach with preservation of its associated perichondrium (Fig. 9.1).

The cartilage–perichondrium graft is prepared by elevating the perichondrium from one side of the cartilage while maintaining its attachment to the other side. The cartilage–perichondrium graft is placed as a medial graft with the elevated perichondrium draping on to the posterior external canal wall for stabilization. The middle ear space and the external auditory canal are packed in a standard way using an absorbable gelatin sponge (Fig. 9.2).

Small central, residual perforations, traumatic perforations, non-healing perforations, and high-risk perforations are included in this group. All these are treated transtympanically

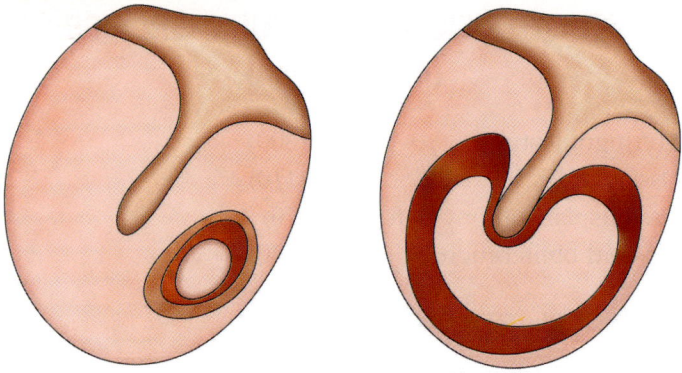

Fig. 9.1. Transtympanic—Island graft myringoplasty

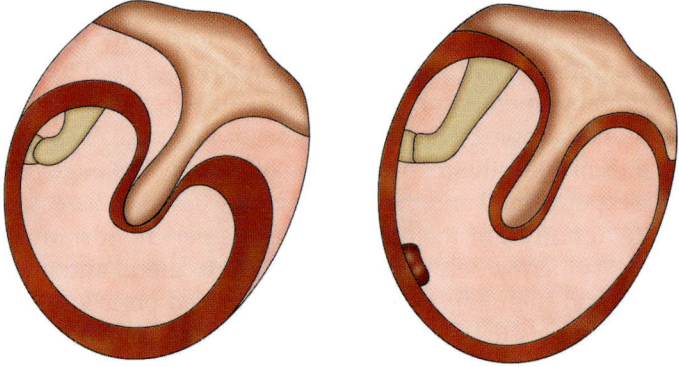

Fig. 9.2. Cartilage–perichondrium composite graft myringoplasty

without raising the tympanomeatal flap. I personally like to close these perforations by using composite cartilage graft technique. The graft is placed through the perforation and spread as inlay graft. No gelfoam is placed in the middle ear. The silastic sheet is placed over the new graft as a support . The graft take is 95 to 96% with excellent hearing.

Postaural or Endaural Approach

The anterior, inferior and posterior perforations are closed by perichondrium-cartilage island flap technique, onlay technique, or butterfly graft techniques.

The middle ear pathology is cleared by doing tympano-mastoid surgery, keeping the entire middle ear clean. The cartilage-perichondrium composite island graft is prepared by cartilage-perichondrial dissection. A small vertical strip of cartilage is cut to accommodate the handle of malleus.

The tympanomeatal flap is raised with the annulus from 12 to 6 o'clock position. The ossicular chain integrity is checked and then prepared graft is placed over the bony annulus and under the handle of malleus. Tympanomeatal flap is replaced back over the canal wall. The silastic sheet is placed over the grafted membrane and a small teracortil wick is kept in the EAC. The routine postoperative care is same as for tympanoplasty. These grafts heal without any problems in 6 weeks time.

The total and subtotal perforations are closed by onlay, butterfly or palisade technique. I prefer the palisade technique in which vertical cartilage strips of 1 mm broad with its perichondrium are arranged parallel to the handle of malleus over the bony annulus and under the handle of malleus.

The tympanomeatal flap is replaced and annulus is fixed with gelfoam pieces. This method is used in total perforation with an intact ossicular chain. In case of defective ossicular chain but with stapes present, the 3 mm broad plates are placed on the bony annulus.

In chronic ET obstruction, the tunnelplasty can be done in the same sitting. This technique prevents retraction, atelactetic and cholesteatoma pockets (Fig. 9.3). Heermann claims excellent hearing results and almost no recurrent perforation.

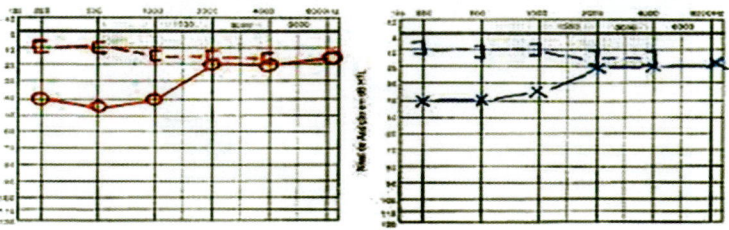

Fig. 9.3. Mild conductive hearing loss in ET obstruction

2. OSSICULOPLASTY (110 CASES)

Endaural or Postaural Approach

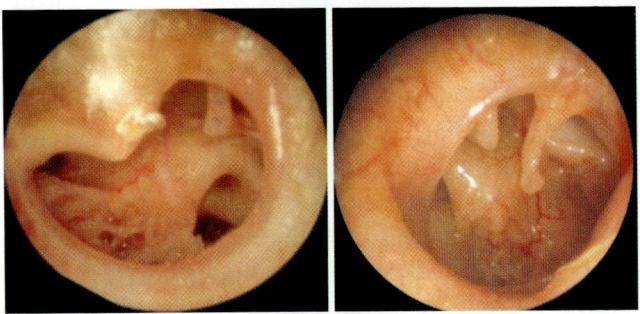

Fig. 9.4. Large central perforations

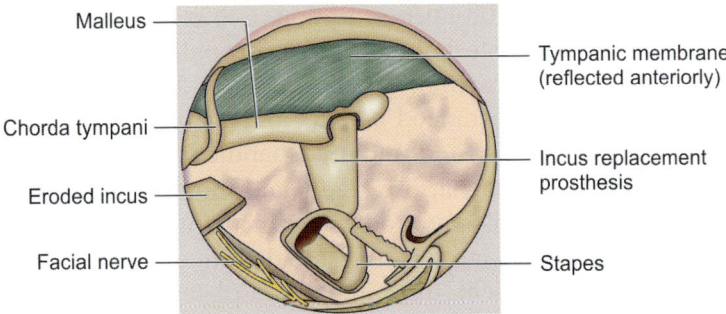

Malleus

Chorda tympani

Eroded incus

Facial nerve

Tympanic membrane
(reflected anteriorly)

Incus replacement
prosthesis

Stapes

Fig. 9.5. Ossicular reconstruction with incus replacement

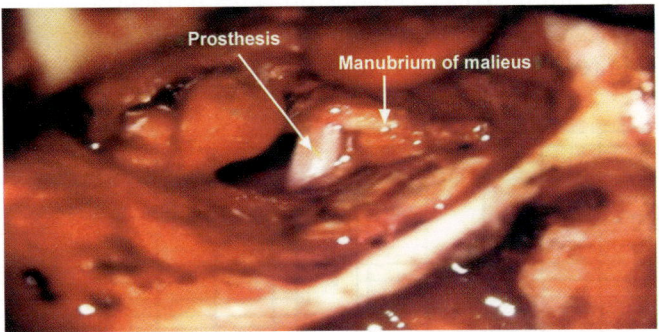

Prosthesis

Manubrium of malleus

Fig. 9.6. Prosthesis has been interposed between the manubrium of the malleus and the capitulum of the stapes (tympanomastoid surgery)

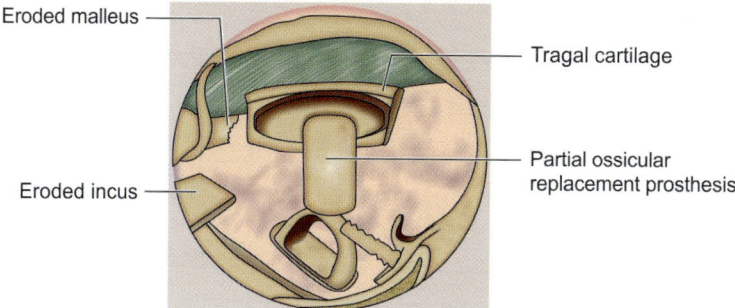

Fig. 9.7. Ossicular reconstruction with PORP with tragal cartilage

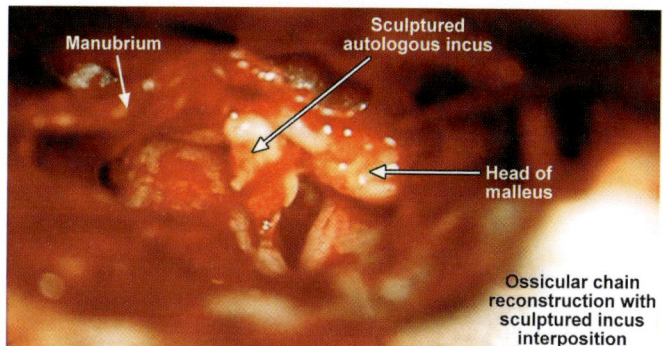

Fig. 9.8. Picture of a left tympanoplasty, the patient's incus was removed, sculptured and interposed between the malleus and the stapes

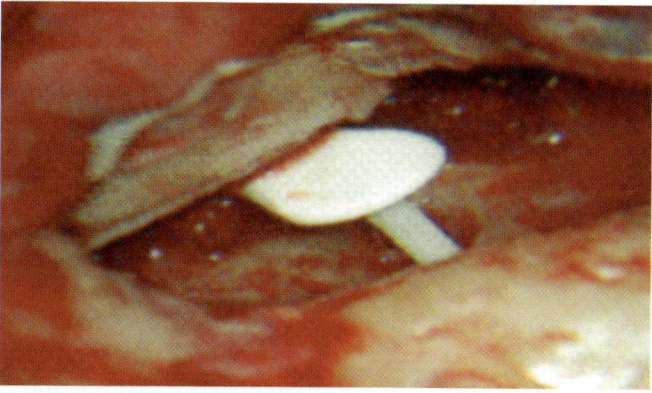

Fig. 9.9. TORP in cartilageplasty (Cartilage in reinforcement of TORPs and PORPs)

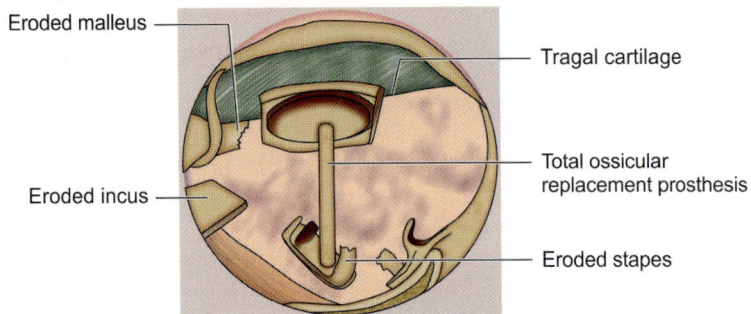

Eroded malleus —
Tragal cartilage —
Eroded incus —
Total ossicular replacement prosthesis —
Eroded stapes —

Fig. 9.10. Ossicular reconstruction with TORP with tragal cartilage

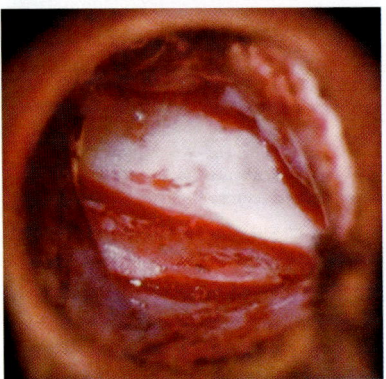

Fig. 9.11. PORP in position clipped, with head plate in posistion

Surgical Technique

In this group, the disease pathlogy is cleared by doing tympano-mastoidectomy and then ossicular reconstruction is done by using various cartilage struts. Incus replacement prosthesis, PORP and TORP creating transformer mechanism and stable ossicular assembly. The reconstruction or reinforcement of TM with cartilage is performed typically with ossiculoplasty to prevent prosthesis extrusion, recurrent retractions, or cholesteatoma pockets. The incidence of necrosis of long process of the incus is the most common ossicular chain pathology. It is three times more common than absence of stapedial arch. Cases are recorded with ossicular disruption following head injury (Anklesaria, Laryngo1963). Consequently, type II ossiculoplasty is the most common procedure in middle ear surgery using cartilage struts of various shapes.

Applications of Different Struts in Ossicular Reconstruction

Ossiculoplasty is done with following methods: (1) Interpositions, (2) transpositions, and (3) pexis.

Interposition refers to placing an ossicle, bony or cartilaginous graft or any other prostheses between the stapes or stapedial arch and the malleus handle or drum making stable assembly.

Transposition refers to procedures in which a cartilage is still attached to its origin (drum) but is transported on to the stapes.

The pexis is of various types, as myringostapediopexy myringoincudopexy, and all kinds of ossicular reconstructions.

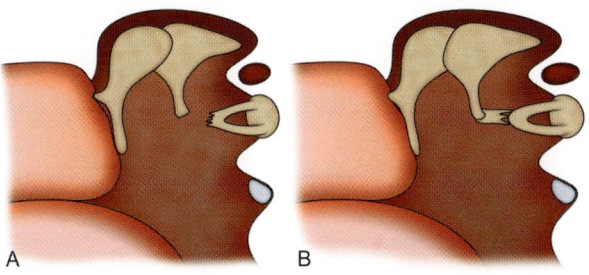

Fig. 9.12A and B. Group I: (A) Incudo-stapedial joint defect, (B) Corrected with cartilage strut

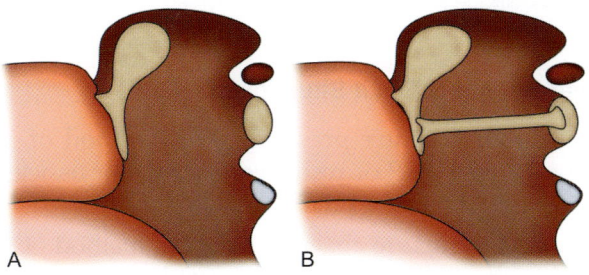

Fig. 9.13A and B. Group III: Incus and stapes superstructured

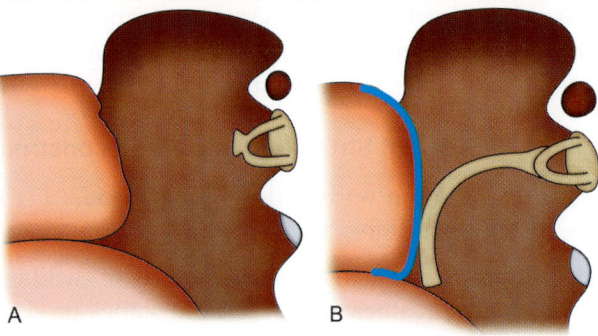

Fig. 9.14A and B. Group IV: (A) Malleus and incus absent or destroyed, (B) Corrected with bow cartilage strut

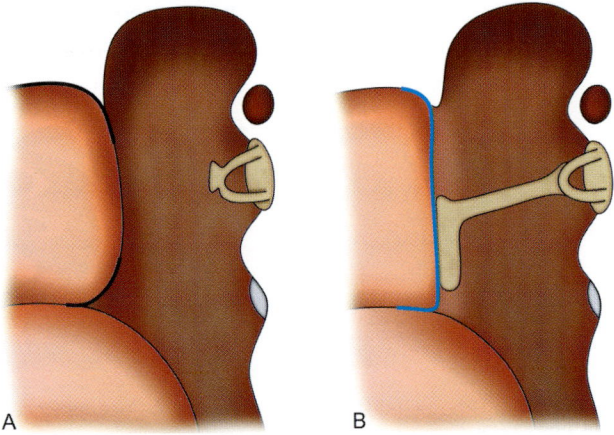

Fig. 9.15A and B. Group IV: (A) Malleus and incus absent or destroyed (B) Corrected with L shaped cartilage strut

Cartilageplasty in Difficult Situations

1. **Stapes superstructure present:** Usual method of reconstruction using PORP or reshaped cartilage or ossicles from malleus—TM to head of the stapes.

2. **Stapes superstructure absent:** The usual method of reconstruction using TORP or replaced cartilage assembly from malleus—TM to stapes footplate.

3. **If malleus is present:** A Y-shaped or T-shaped cartilage from malleus to footplate can be used.

4. **If malleus is absent:** Two-cartilage technique is used. The first cartilage arches from a depression drilled in the inferior annulus to the footplate. The second cartilage is from the superior annulus to a small depression made in the first cartilage for pressure contact.

5. **If the lenticular process of incus is necrosed:** A cartilage extending from the inferior annulus fitting between the long process and the stapes is used.

6. **If the end of long process of the incus is slightly eroded,** it can be reinforced by a cartilage placed from the inferior annulus to the incudo-stapedial joint.

7. **If the malleus handle is necrosed** as in total perforation, a cartilage of Y-shaped from the inferior annulus to incudo-stapedial joint is reconstructed.

3. OSSIOUSPLASTY (100 CASES) (RECONSTRUCTION OF BONY DEFECTS)

Sr. no.	Lesion	Cases	%
1.	Attic	50	50
2.	PSQ	33	30
3.	PCW	10	10
4.	ET	10	10
	Total	**100**	**100**

In this group, the bony defects in the attic, posterosuperior quadrant, posterior canal wall; and the annular defects caused by extensive cholesteatoma are reconstructed. In the first instance, the complete middle ear pathology should be cleared by tympanomastoid surgery and the defects are reconstructed by canalplasty using conchal cartilage or tragal cartilage perichondrium composite grafts.

The attic defects are healed very nicely within six weeks. The PSQ defects are also treated in the same way and reconstructed. Here conchal cartilage would be an ideal graft material used. The defects in bony annulus can be reconstructed by natural angle of tragal perichondrium which is a perfect fit for the annulus. The ET defects are reconstructed by tunnelplasty. The advantages of this cartilageplasty are to mould the defective anatomy into normal anatomy of ME.

The results are very gratifying and is about **84%.**

4. MASTOID OBLITERATION (120 CASES)

Indications for Mastoid Obliteration

1. Canal wall-down mastoidectomy.
2. Chronic otorrhoea, non-healing mastoid bowl.
3. Translabyrinthine acoustic neuroma resection.
4. CSF leak.
5. Extensive temporal bone trauma.
6. Temporal bone malignancy.
7. Cochlear implantation in CSOM

Relative Contraindication

Persistent Active Disease (Malignancy)

The concept of mastoid obliteration was first introduced in 1911 by Mosher to promote the healing of a mastoidectomy defect. The vast majority of obliteration techniques consist of either local flaps (muscle, periosteum and fascia) or free grafts (cartilage, bone, hydroxyapatite). Mosher, Kish and Rombo, Popper and Pulva flaps were popular. Other materials being used are bone pate, fat, diced cartilage and fascia, bone chips and ceramic materials.

We have used consistently tragal cartilage with superiorly based temporalis swing to obliterate the mastoid cavities and found to be very satisfactory.

Autogenous tragal cartilage or conchal cartilage was introduced in reconstructive tympanoplasty by Utech (1961),

Goodhill (1961), Gilford (1961), Farrior (1962), Heermann (1963), Heermann and Heermann (1964), and Mccleve (1969).

Obliteration is done in both canal wall down and canal wall up mastoidectomy. In modern obliteration of the mastoid cavity, the posterior canal wall is always reconstructed along with wide meatoplasty. Autogenous cartilage was the only obliteration material used by Heermann over many years.

Tragal and conchal cartilages are cut with their peri-chondrium and placed on the exposed cavity walls. The palisade technique with intact perichondrium prevents ingrowths of epidermis through the interstices of the cartilage. Tragal cartilage or conchal cartilage is used for partial obliteration of supralabyrinthine space and attic space and it is also used in attic wall reconstruction.

Surgical Procedure

The old radical and modified radical cavities are reconstructed with cartilage perichondrium grafts with maximum lowering of facial ridge to the level of facial nerve. It is absolutely essential that the cavities are drilled effectively and saucerized using cutting and diamond burrs. No ridges or cavities to be seen after complete cavity saucerization. The posterior canal wall is reconstructed by conchal cartilage. The anterior canal bulge should be adequately treated by canalplasty and then the mastoid cavity is obliterated by palisade technique **(palis-adeplasty).** Temporalis muscle with its fascia is used in cavity obliteration by swing technique covering the entire cavity. It is absolutely essential that a wide meatoplasty is created for postoperative cavity toilet.

The surgical intervention involved partial mastoid oblitera-tion (Fig. 9.16) and restoration of the middle ear space by use of cartilage reconstruction of the tympanic membrane. Ossicular reconstruction was achieved with either a partial or total ossicular replacement prosthesis. Because this technique involved contouring the mastoid cavity, the problems that usually occur, such as drainage or debris collection, were alleviated. In addition, re-establishment of the middle ear space often restored hearing. A completely dry cavity was achieved

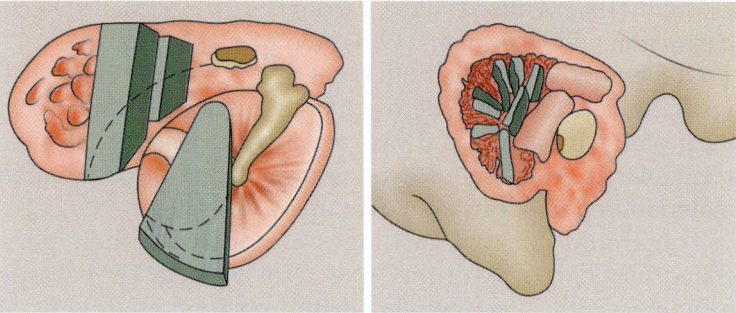

Fig. 9.16. Mastoid obliteration

in 18 of 20 patients. An overall statistically significant improvement in hearing (P <0.05) was obtained, with the mean pure-tone average air-bone gap decreasing to 16.1 dB from 36.5 dB. This technique has proven to be a useful adjunct in the surgical management of the chronically draining cavity.

Postoperative Treatment

At 1 to 2 weeks postoperative surgery, the packing material of gelfoam and antibiotic ointment is completely suctioned from external canal. Antibiotic steroid-containing eardrops are used for additional 2 weeks to clear the ear of residual ointment and gelfoam which will prevent granulations and fibrosis. All adult patients are instructed to start Valsalva manoeuvre. Post-operative audiogram is obtained 6 to 8 weeks later. All patients are given antibiotics, antihistaminics and anti-inflammatory drugs for further six weeks along with local steroidal drops.

Postoperative Results of Cartilage Tympanoplasty

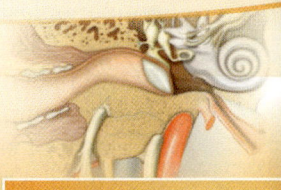

10

1. MYRINGOPLASTY GROUP: TOTAL 300 CASES

Transcanal-transtympanic myringoplasty was done in **72** cases, where only perichondrium was used. The onlay grafting was done in 100 cases, and underlay grafting was done in 128 cases. In this group, the graft take rate was **96%** and failure rate was **4%** due to infection, displacement of graft. The hearing gain with SRT was achieved within 15dB of BC. The failed cases had to undergo revision myringoplasty. The follow-up was achieved in 75% of the cases for over 3 years.

Successful closure occurred in 96%. The only independent factor to determine this success rate was the preoperative ABG. As for ABG gain it significantly increased from 15.91 to 8.82 dB postoperatively with a mean gain of 7.09 dB. The statistically important factors affecting this ABG gain was found to be the preoperative ABG followed by perforation size.

2. OSSICULOPLASTY GROUP: TOTAL 110 CASES

These cases were done by underlay and overlay technique for reconstructing the tympanic membrane and ossicular chain with various combinations of different composite cartilage-perichondrium struts and some cases with TORP and PORP. The various incudo-stapedial, malleo-stapes and malleo-footplate assembly were performed. In this group, the success rate was **84%** and failure rate was **16%.** The failures were due to infection, displacement of prosthesis and extrusion of the graft. The results were better in type III than type II tympanoplasty. The audiometric thresholds by SRT methods revealed 15 to 20 dB AB closure. The follow-up was achieved in 70% of patients for 3 to 5 years, failed cases were subjected for revision tympanoplasty with ossicular reconstruction. Extrusion of plastic or ceramic implants is a significant cause of failure in ossiculoplasty for chronic ear disease. The composite tragal cartilage and perichondrial autograft compared to cartilage or bone paste between the graft and tympanic membrane. At 5 years, there were no extrusions in the group with the composite graft ($n= 90$) and 20 extrusions in the cartilage/bone paste group ($n= 20$) ($P= 0.02$). The mean average air-bone gap was significantly better for the composite grafts at 5 years (15 dB vs 24 dB) ($P < 0.05$). Extrusions were eliminated and hearing results better at 5 years using the composite graft. We recommend the composite cartilage-perichondrium grafts in ossicular reconstruction which has excellent results.

3. OSSIOUSPLASTY GROUP:70 CASES (BONY DEFECTS RECONSTRUCTION)

Bony defects of attic, PSQ and bony annulus were reconstructed with cartilage-perichondrium plates. The defects due to cholesteatoma, or surgical trauma were first removed by radical surgery clearing all the disease entity from attic additus, posterior canal wall and PSQ region and then the graftings were done using tragal cartilage or conchal cartilage with its perichondrium attached. For posterior canal wall, the ideal graft was conchal cartilage which fitted in the defect of the posterior canal wall. Large defects were treated with composite grafts. The bony annulus was reconstructed with natural angle of perichondrium. This is the exact fit for missing bony annulus. The defects healed in 4 to 6 weeks time without any postoperative complications. By 30 and 70 degrees angle endoscopes, special attention was paid to the facial recess and sinus tympani for disease clearance. The ossiousplasty group achieved **75%** success rate and **25%** were failures which were again subjected for revision tympanoplasty.

4. MASTOID OBLITERATION GROUP: TOTAL 120 CASES

All mastoid cavities were vigorously treated with oto-microscopic suction clearance for 4 to 6 weeks. Along with systemic antibiotics and local steroidal and antifungal ear drops until the cavities were dry enough to undergo obliteration procedures. The cavities were drilled with cutting and diamond burrs and all residual disease were cleared. I personally like to use cartilage-perichondrium palisadeplasty for obliteration of the cavities.

The plates of cartilage-perichondrium were cut and arranged either horizontal or vertical fashion to cover the cavity and temporalis muscle swing with its fascia is placed in the cavity. The cavities were re-epithelialised well and achieved **70%** success rate. The modified radical cavities were transformed into radical cavities with type III tympanoplasties. In this series the failure rate was **25%** which was due to recurrent infection and poor follow-ups. The cartilage in obliteration of the mastoid cavity will not change the shape after any fibrosis. The problems of mastoid cavities are still unsolved and needs further definite and curative treatment.

Table 10.1: Grouping of middle ear surgery

Sr.no	Group	Success	Failure
1.	Myringoplasty group	96%	4%
2.	Ossiculoplasty group	84%	16%
3.	Ossiousplasty group	75%	25%
4.	Mastoid obliteration group	70%	30%

POSTOPERATIVE RESULTS OF PRIMARY CARTILAGEPLASTY

The goals of a successful tympanoplasty procedure are creation of an intact and mobile tympanic membrane, mucolised and aerated middle ear and mobile ossicular conductive apparatus. Cartilage has shown promise as a graft material to close perforations in the tympanic membrane (TM), particularly in cases of advanced middle ear pathology. Although it is similar to fascia, its more rigid quality tends to resist resorption and retraction. However, it is this rigid quality that has led many to anticipate a significant conductive hearing loss when using cartilage to reconstruct the TM. Because little has been reported in the literature comparing hearing results using cartilage with other grafting materials.

Both series of cartilage and fascia had undergone type I tympanoplasty, and the middle ear pathology was considered to be similar between the two groups. TM closure was achieved in all 300 patients undergoing cartilage reconstruction, but in 60 patients undergoing fascia reconstruction had a recurrent perforation during the follow-up period (approximately 1 year). The average pre- and postoperative pure-tone average air-bone gap (PTA-ABG) was 21.1 dB and 6.8 dB for the cartilage group and 17.9 dB and 7.7 dB for the perichondrium group, respectively. These gains in hearing were statistically significant (P < 0.001 in each case), but there was no statistically significant difference in hearing results between the two groups. Analysis of the PTA-ABG as a function of percentage of TM reconstructed showed no statistically significant difference in hearing results due to percentage of cartilage used. These results indicate that cartilage tympanoplasty offers the possibility of a rigorous TM reconstruction with excellent postoperative hearing results.

Patients' ages ranged from 18 to 60 years (mean 39). Mean postoperative follow-up was 60 months. Graft-take was achieved in 300 patients (96.35%). In the two failures (revision surgery), a marginal perforation and a lateralization of the graft occurred. There were no immediate postoperative complications such as wound infection, haematoma, sensorineural hearing loss or facial nerve injury.

At follow-up, 10% who underwent a second-stage procedure for cholesteatoma were found to have limited residual disease, which was treated successfully. Recurrent cholesteatoma was observed in 10 cases. The overall mean preoperative PTA-ABG was 43.79 ±7.07 dB, whereas the postoperative (1 year after surgery) PTA-ABG was 10.43 ±5.25 dB (p <0.0001). A statistically significant improvement was observed up to 5 years after surgery.

The results of the present study suggest that cartilage is a good grafting material, in fact it is easily accessible, easy to fashion, resistant to negative middle ear pressures, stable (particularly in cases lacking fibrous annulus), sufficiently elastic for good sound conduction, well tolerated, and resistant to resorption.

Furthermore, cartilage prevents extrusion of the prosthesis, when this is used for ossicular reconstruction, and above all, it does not involve additional costs. A potential drawback of this procedure is the graft opacity, as it may be more difficult to detect eventual residual/recurrent cholesteatoma. However, also the fascia is often not transparent. In our study, we observed 8% rate of reperforation.

These results demonstrate that hearing results after cartilage tympanoplasty are comparable to those after temporalis fascia tympanoplasty. Therefore, when indicated, a cartilage–perichondrium graft can be used to reconstruct or strengthen a large portion of the tympanic membrane without fear of impairing hearing. It is our practice to size the graft slightly larger than the atelectatic portion of the tympanic membrane.

COMPLICATIONS OF CARTILAGE TYMPANOPLASTY

During the study period, we have not seen major complications apart from usual tympanoplasty complications which can be corrected by revision surgery.

1. Infection
2. Displacement of graft

Table 10.2: Poor results in cartilageplasty

Sr. no	Causes	Cases	%
1	Displacement	12	2
2	Fibrosis	10	1.6
3	Absorption	6	1
4	Infection	8	1.3
Total		36	6

3. Displacement of cartilage studs (ossiculoplasty)
4. Adhesive changes
5. Conductive hearing loss

THE FATE OF THE CARTILAGE GRAFT IN TYMPANOPLASTY

Autograft tragal cartilages and preserved homograft nasal septal cartilages removed from revision tympanoplasty were examined with histologic and histochemical stains. The implanted cartilage remained in the middle ear from 6 to 18 months without significant inflammatory reaction or evidence of resorption. It appears that the implanted cartilages removed from tympanoplasty have been well tolerated in the middle ear space.

The otological researches on cartilage grafts evoke very little cellular response and demonstrate that the presence of an intact and established blood supply of the host area contributes to and hastens the union (Davidson-1959). However, the issue on the fate of the cartilage is still controversial. The fate of the cartilage has not yet been investigated.

Another study by Steinbach and Pusalkar (1981) for cartilage columella or struts in ossiculoplasty demonstrated that because of fibrosis of the cartilage the columellae becomes soft, which changes the shape and function. The transmission of vibrations is inadequate, resulting in hearing loss. Therefore, if the full thickness cartilage plates (2 × 2 mm) with perichondrium interposed between the stapes head then eardrum functions well and does not suffer change of shape. In this, extrusion is very rare.

In our study, we have used four techniques as cartilage perichondrium composite island graft, butterfly graft, palisade graft, and schield graft and found grafts were well survived on long-term basis with follow-up of 3 to 5 years. The fate of the graft is dependent on its nourishment. The nourishment of cartilage is achieved by diffusion with the help of perichondrium. For this reason, the nourishment of the graft will be optimal, if the cartilage graft is covered on both sides with perichondrium. The poor nourishment as a poor covering of the perichondrium may cause late changes in the graft, such as necrosis and perforations of the reconstructed eardrum.

THE IMPORTANT TIPS FOR SUCCESSFUL CARTILAGE TYMPANOPLASTY

1. Surgical intervention should be as atraumatic as possible both with the graft and the donor place.
2. Use graft with perichondrium covering on both sides.
3. Provide good conditions for the epithelialization of both sides of the cartilage graft.
4. Save the the keratinized squamous epithelium of the eardrum remnant for outer covering of the cartilage with the epithelium.
5. In onlay techniques, the cartilage graft is placed on the denuded edge of the lamina propria and the epithelium is replaced on to the perichondrium or close to it.
6. In inlay techniques, epithelialization of the outer side of the cartilage is easy, if the graft is in close contact with the undersurface of the eardrum.
7. The covering of the undersurface of the cartilage graft should be promoted by scarification or removal of edge of the perforation.
8. The application of evicel (fibrin sealant by Johnson & Johnson) after completion of grafting procedure will be an added advantage in successful cartilage tympanoplasty.

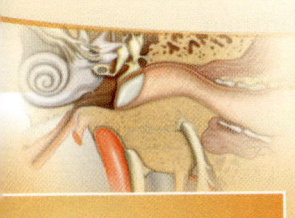

Efficasy of Evicel
(Fibrin Sealant—Human)
In Composite Cartilage
Graft Myringoplasty
(Prospective Study)

11

INTRODUCTION

Fibrin sealant has been used for many years and has a wide range of clinical applications for suture support, tissue adhesion, and haemostasis. Fibrin sealant imitates the final phase of the blood coagulation process. Fibrinogen is converted to fibrin on a tissue surface by the action of thrombin, which is then cross-linked by factor XIIIa, creating a mechanically stable fibrin network. This fibrin network is thought to reduce the amount of postoperative bleeding by sealing capillary vessels and enabling raw operative surfaces of cartilage graft to adhere. The potential advantages of the use of such substances include prevention of haematoma, reduction in surgical time, reduction in flap oedema, and shorter recovery time and excellent healing. The physiologic mechanism that creates fibrin sealant was first described by Morawitz in 1905.

We have reviewed the world literature to find out if any study in micro-ear surgery is done but could find very few studies confirming the role of evicel. Ours is the first pilot study to know the efficacy of evicel sealant in reconstructive tympanoplasty. Fibrin glue was originally described in 1970 and is formed by polymerizing fibrinogen with thrombin and calcium. It was originally prepared using donor plasma; however, because of the low concentration of fibrinogen in plasma, the stability and quality of the fibrin glue were low. Commercially, pretreated fibrin sealant products were developed to increase the efficacy of forming a stable clot. These products are heat treated, which greatly reduces the risk of disease transmission. The fibrin sealant and delivery system are easy to store and rapid to construct, and, therefore, have enjoyed some use in reconstructive tympanoplasty and cosmetic surgery.

Fibrin sealant (human) (Evicel; Johnson and Johnson–Wound Management, Somerville, New Jersey) is a plasma cryopreci-pitate-based sealant that consists of two components: (1) bio-logical active component–2 (BAC2), also called human clottable protein, which consists predominantly of fibrinogen and (2) thrombin. BAC2, a concentrated solution of clottable plasma proteins, consists mainly of fibrinogen and other proteins. The thrombin solution contains highly purified human thrombin and calcium chloride for activation of clotting of the final combined product. Thrombin is a highly specific protease that transforms the fibrinogen contained in BAC2 into fibrin. It is indicated as supportive treatment in patients undergoing reconstructive tympanoplasty.

ABOUT EVICEL SEALANT

- Thaws within 10 minutes at 37°C (and must not be kept at this temperature for longer than 10 minutes); within 1 hour at 20°C to 25°C (room temperature); or within 1 day at 2°C to 8°C (refrigerator). Once thawed, EVICEL® must not be refrozen. Once at room temperature, EVICEL® must not be refrigerated.

- All-human formulation–EVICEL® fibrin sealant does not contain aprotinin or bovine derivatives and does not expose patients to the risks associated with aprotinin.

- Multiple, clog-resistant tip options—standard 6 cm tip or 35 cm rigid or 45 cm flexible tip.

Important Risk Information

- Do not inject directly into the circulatory system. Intra-vascular application of EVICEL® may result in life-threatening thromboembolic events.

- Do not use in individuals known to have anaphylactic or severe systemic reaction to human blood products.
- Do not use for the treatment of severe or brisk arterial bleeding.

Most common adverse events reported in clinical trials (=5%) are bradycardia, nausea, hypokalaemia, insomnia, hypotension, pyrexia, graft infection, vascular graft occlusion, peripheral oedema, and constipation.

PREPARATION OF EVICEL SEALANT

Evicel is provided as a single-use human surgical sealant kit consisting of 2 packages, the first containing 1 vial each of frozen sterile solutions of BAC2 (biological active componant 2) and thrombin and the second containing the sterile application device (Fig. 11.1). It is the only totally human protein–derived, bovine-free fibrin sealant commercially available in the United States. The unit cost for 2 ml of fibrin sealant plus the applicator is $200 (₹ 12000). The vials are stored in a freezer; when removed and thawed, they are stable for 24 hours. The vials are readily thawed in 5 minutes without the use of a rapid-warming device. After the BAC2 and thrombin solutions are thawed, they are drawn into a unique trilumenal (2 syringe lumens and 1 air lumen for spraying) catheter application device (Fig. 11.2). As the plungers are depressed simultaneously, the solutions are mixed by the applicator and sprayed into the operative site.

The applicator gently sprays the fibrin sealant into the operative wound as a thin layer and, therefore, allows a relatively small volume (1 ml) of sealant to be delivered evenly

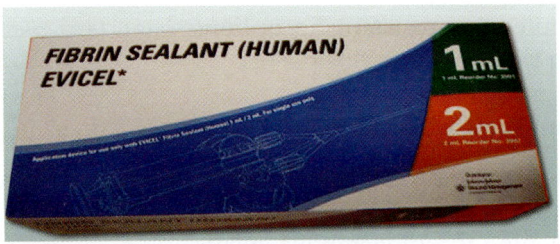

Fig. 11.1. Evicel sealant pack of two bulbs of one cc each

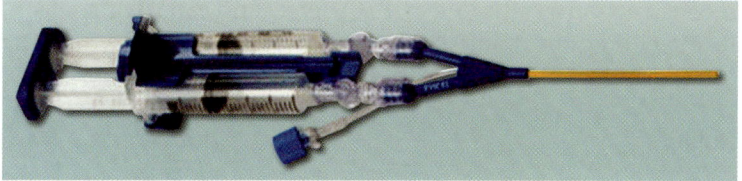

Fig. 11.2. Evicel applicator syrinege

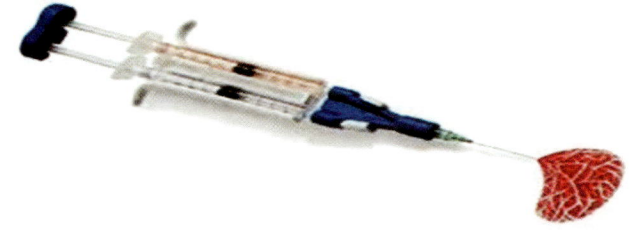

Fig. 11.3. Tissue surface application of evicel by triluminal syrinege over new graft

(Fig. 11.3). The solutions mix as they exit the catheter during administration, are applied topically by dripping and once applied are transparent. The reconstituted preparation mimics the final steps in physiologic coagulation. Fibrinogen is converted to fibrin on the wound surface in presence of calcium ions by the actions of thrombin and factor XIII, all derived from human plasma. A stable cross-linked fibrin clot is formed over the neotympanum.

Recently, we have done 50 cases of type one tympanoplasties with inlay composite cartilage graft. After the surgical procedure is over, the evicel (1 ml) solution is applied over the surface of the graft material by the evicel triluminal applicator and it was kept for over 3 to 5 minutes to form a solid layer over the neotympanum. So far 50 casers being treated with this technique and found to be excellent in graft take up (98%) and without medialization or lateralization. No complications encountered during evicel application. Graft take was 98% postoperatively. More study will be required for its efficacy in reconstructive tympanoplasty. We plan to do more cases with varied middle ear pathology like ossiculoplasty, ossiousplasty (bony defect reconstruction as attic defect, PSQ defect and canal wall defect). Its effect on graft fixing is very encouraging which inspired us to take up this study in middle ear reconstruction.

Results

- The results were evaluated in the form of graft uptake, hearing outcome and complications.
- Healed neotympanic membrane, which moves on seigelization was taken as successful graft take-up, while any

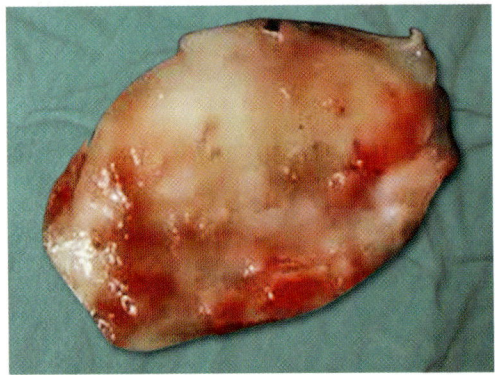

Fig. 11.4. Layer of evicel application over the cartilage–perichondrium graft

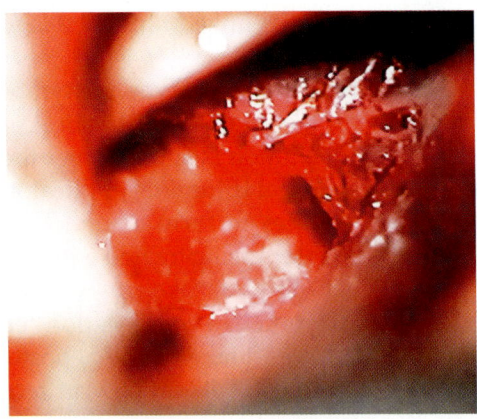

Fig. 11.5. Intraoperative evicel

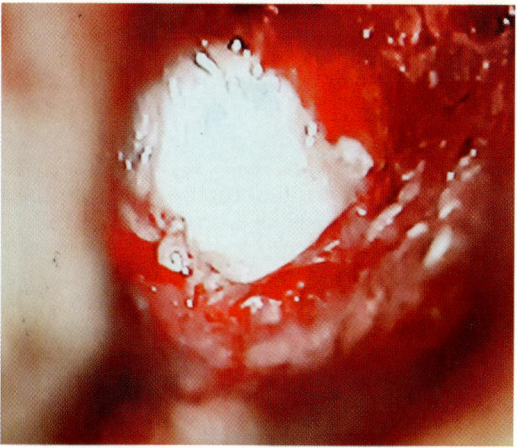

Fig. 11.6. Postoperative evicel—1 week

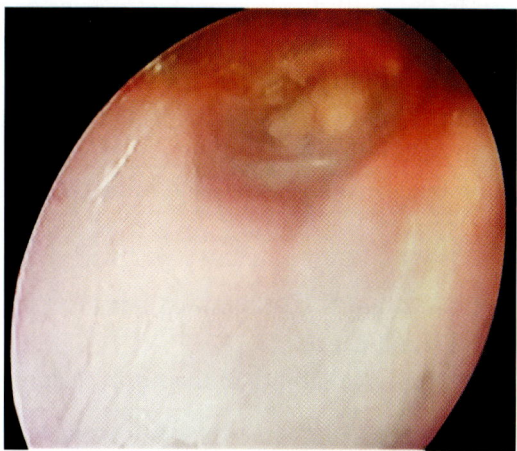

Fig. 11.7. Postoperative evicel—6 weeks

residual perforations or retraction of neotympanum were taken as failures.

- Postoperative and preoperative pure-tone audiograms were compared. Hearing gain and mean residual gaps were evaluated in speech frequencies of 500, 1000, and 2000 Hz.

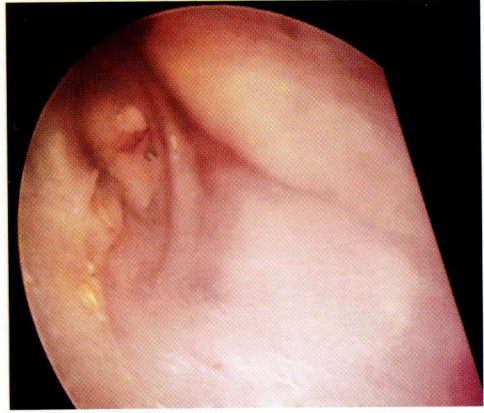

Fig. 11.8. Postoperative evicel—8 weeks

Advantages

- Reduction in the graft displacement as a cause of failure.
- Ease of use. Comes with the application device and is easy to set up and ready to use.
- Works on all types of grafts so your primary surgery does not need any alterations.
- Application takes just an extra few minutes at the end of the surgery.

Drawbacks

- Need for a longer study with more number of cases to prove its statistical significance.
- Affordability and availability of the fibrin sealant.

To Summurize

- A failure rate of around 10% for a type I tympanoplasty is still high by today's standards.
- The pilot study shows promising results.
- Encourage ENT surgeons to use a fibrin sealant and publish your results and feedback regarding the same.

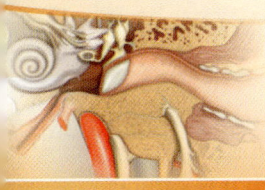

Discussion

12

For many years, the so-called conservative methods of radical and modified radical operations (Barany, Bondy, Citell, Heerman, Stacke) were done in the clearance of disease but none of these proved better. At later dates, Farrior, House, Lempert, and Morrison added some minor variations in the technique of reconstructive tympanoplasty but still could not achieve the better results because the recurrence rate was very high. To modify these techniques, Victor Goodhill, Heermann and Heerman demonstrated their new technique using tragal cartilage which prevented the recurrence of the cholesteatoma and gained high success rates.

First described in 1952 by Wullstein and Zöllner, tympanoplasty is the mainstay for tympanic membrane reconstruction. Grafting materials initially were of epidermal origin, and later various mesenchymal tissues, including vein, fascia, perichondrium, and periosteum, were used. Today fascia of the temporalis muscle is the most frequently used material for tympanoplasty. Cartilage was first used in middle ear surgery for ossicular chain reconstruction in 1958 by Jansen. In 1963, Salen and Jansen first reported the use of cartilage composite grafts for tympanic membrane reconstruction.

Since the first description of tympanoplasty, clinicians have attempted to reduce the frequency of complications such as recurrent tympanic membrane retraction and cholesteatoma. The selection of surgical technique is directed by the pathology encountered. In cases of severe tympanic membrane retraction, atelectasis, cholesteatoma, or perforation in the setting of Eustachian tube dysfunction, cartilage tympanoplasty has been shown to be a safe alternative to temporalis fascia or peri-chondrium grafting.

Cartilage has shown promise as a graft material to close perforations in the tympanic membrane (TM), particularly in cases of advanced middle ear pathology. Although it is similar to fascia, its more rigid quality tends to resist resorption and retraction. However, it is this rigid quality that has led many to anticipate a significant conductive hearing loss when using cartilage to reconstruct the TM. Because little has been reported in the literature comparing hearing results using cartilage with results using other grafting materials, this retrospective study was conducted to compare the hearing results of patients with cartilage tympanoplasty with results in patients who underwent revision tympanoplasty using perichondrium and fascia.

With changing trends, even the search for an ideal reconstructive material. "**The graft**" has undergone many phases starting from materials like pig's bladder mucosa to fascia grafts and from ceramics to plastipores. Amongst all these, emerged Victor Goodhill's introduction of tragal cartilage and perichondrium for the repair of the tympanic membrane as well as ossicles in 1962. Numerous studies carried out have proved that tragal cartilage and perichondrium is a valuable grafting material. Various other materials include autografts, plastic materials, wire prosthesis, plastipores, ceramics, etc. The literature review revealed "Every graft material has its own drawbacks".

Autografts are found to be excellent in tympanoplasties. In benign type of middle ear pathology, tympanic membrane and ossicles may be affected due to hyperaemic process in chronic inflammation (Sade). In case of adhesive otitis, the drum may be adherent and ossicles may not be found to be suitable to repose, due to surrounding fibrosis.

In tympanosclerosis, plaques can be seen on the drum and in some cases incudomalleolar fixation was seen in attic region. The ossicles were partly destroyed and sometimes too brittle. The reduction in blood supply may be the possible cause. In case of cholesteatoma, ossicles show destruction or erosion due to pressure necrosis, enzyme activity or inflammatory changes in middle ear and even the posterosuperior canal wall may be eroded. Cholesteatoma matrix may also be found in remnant of bone. Hence, the use of autografts ossicles remains controversial.

In the absence or overtly destroyed autograft, **homograft ossicles** are an alternative. Due to lack of proper facilities for preservation of homograft, and the fear of spread of infectious diseases, their use in our country remains impracticable.

Cortical bone chips have been used to bridge small gaps in the chain but they tend to resorb in time (Pukec and Sheehy). **Polythene grafts** recommended at one time are not satisfactory. Foreign body reaction results in extrusion. Osteolytic reaction to polythene resulted in necrosis of adjacent ossicles and failure (Pulec and Sheehy). **Wire prosthesis** also has the risk of extrusion and has the problem to obtain a secure attachment to a mobile stapes footplate. **Ceramics, plastipore and other synthetic materials** again are at risk of extrusion or are costly to use.

The objective of the study was to assess the efficacy of cartilage perichondrium for, functional capacity in restoring hearing, its mechanical survival, its extrusion rate, and its functional integrity in tympanomastoid reconstruction. The study was divided into four groups as myringoplasty, ossiculoplasty, ossiousplasty (bony defects) and mastoid obliteration. The various techniques of reconstruction are discussed with their advantages and disadvantages. The general impression from the literature, however, is that graft survival is very similar to fascia.

The one significant point is revealed from the study that in revision surgery the ideal graft material is cartilage-perichondrium which prevents recurrence of cholesteatoma, posterior retractions, atelectasis and tympanosclerosis. The tragal cartilage is typically slightly less than 1 mm thick and, therefore, is used as a full-thickness graft. Using the Doppler interferometer, Zahnert suggested a slight acoustic benefit by thinning the cartilage to 0.5 mm by cartilage slicer, but this advantage is offset by the curling of the graft. Therefore, since our hearing results have been good, we recommend full-thickness grafts for cartilage reconstruction of the eardrum.

In this study, use of cartilage and perichondrium for myringoplasty and tympanoplasty shows some distinct advantages. It is easily accessible in middle ear surgery and is a valuable source of autograft material for drum and ossicular substitution. In case of missing auto-ossicles. Cartilage is a good alternative rigid material, avoiding complications of using other materials. The tragus is usually of adequate stiffness in adults. The cartilage can be moulded in any size or shape for ossiculoplasty.

Cartilage grafts provide good area of contact of new chain with drum or neodrum. Type III tympanoplasty has contact of head of stapes with new drum, which is inadequate for the lever ratio. Augmentation of head of stapes with auto-ossicle or bone chip also may have the same problem.

The difference in surface area between the normal pars tensa and stapes footplate results in concentration of sound energy during its transmission through middle ear space. It is, therefore, important that surface area and compliance of membrane tensa be as near normal as possible (Smyth). This area ratio is well maintained with use of L-shaped graft when handle of malleus is missing. The cartilage graft also restores the middle ear volume thus following the principle of ossicular chain reconstruction to provide air-containing middle ear space.

Another principle of reconstructive surgery is to provide the chain with adequate stiffness and stability and enough tension. This will provide the continuity and will also prevent damping of vibrations. The new ossicular chain with use of tragal cartilage assures mobility when used under adequate tension. This condition is easily fulfilled when handle of malleus is intact. In its absence, the natural curvature and elasticity of tragal cartilage can be used to provide adequate tension. At the same time, this new chain does not become bulky, avoiding complications due to pressure on the footplate of stapes.

Cartilage does not adhere to bone (Pulec and Sheehy) and so it permits motion even when in contact with bony surface

(Proctor and Proctor). The functional viability of the cartilage has been proved by excellent results 3 years postoperatively (Harris and Goodhill). Our study presents a maximum follow-up 10 years with good results. The cases where second look surgery was needed showed evidence of lining of mucous membrane covering the cartilage graft (Don and Linthicum). Evidence of inflammatory reaction was noticed by Steinbach and Pusalkar in some cases, where they had removed the cartilage used in earlier operation.

Biological features of cartilage (Gray) are low antigenicity of its matrix, relatively low vascularity and isolation of chondrocytes in lacunae. These features aid the use of cartilage for transplantation without evoking a marked immune response. Hence, it is better tolerated. **High tensile strength and low metabolic rate are the most important properties of cartilage which assure functional viability**. The molecular architecture of cartilage provides it the compression resisting capacity (Gray). The cartilage removed is also useful in tympanoplasty for other purposes. It can be used for reconstructing or closing the defects in the attic and canal wall. Cartilage rim can also be used to form the lacking tympanic annulus.

This study includes the use of cartilage and perichondrium of reconstructive ear surgery of various types. A total of 600 patients in whom cartilage and perichondrium were used for tympanic membrane reconstruction were studied. Out of 600 cases, 450 cases were primary and 150 cases were revision. Majority of the cases were young adults between age groups of 15–40 years. The main complaint of patients was otorrhoea and deafness. This was so especially in patients with bilateral diseased cases. The ear with more serious pathology or worse level of hearing was selected for surgery. Local anaesthesia with sedation was preferred. Apprehensive adults were operated under general anaesthesia. The use of local anaesthesia with adrenaline showed the advantages of a dry operative field because of better haemostasis. This also avoids formation of adhesions postoperatively. Post-aural and end-aural approaches were used for tympanoplasty and endomeatal approach was used in some cases of myringoplasty. In very small central residual and traumatic perforations, transcanal-transtympanic approach was used (without raising the tympanomeatal flap) in reconstruction of eardrum.

The type of pathology observed during the study was perforations, adhesive otitis media, tympanosclerosis, retraction pockets, and cholesteatoma. It was our observation that biological materials, like cartilage, perichondrium fascia or ossicles, etc., are much better than non-biological materials in reconstructive tympanoplasty. The survival rate of cartilage graft is much better than the non-biological materials. It is also revealed that the extrusion rate of cartilage is very minimum (1.19%) as compared to other grafts.

In mastoid cavity obliterations, the palisade grafting gave excellent results in gaining dry cavities in 75% of the cases. The radical cavities were reduced in size either by reconstruction of the posterior meatal wall with cartilage or by obliteration with cartilage perichondrium and covered with two strips of meatal wall skin. Chronic Eustachain tube obstruction was corrected by tunnelplasty and improved good aeration. The cartilage bridge over the promontory and hypotympanum assures the proper contact with stapes and prevents adhesions with promontory. In CAT procedures, the recurrence of choles-teatoma from facial recess and sinus tympani could be prevented by incorporating the composite tragal perichondrium grafts. In all cases of CAT, we recommend the use of angled endoscopes to rule out the sinus and facial recess hidden pathology. It is also important that cartilage plays a crucial role in reinforcement of TM in conjunction with ossiculoplasty, using TORP and PORP procedures.

In palisade cartilage plasty, fragments were placed parallel to the manubrium of the malleus in type I tympanoplasty and in type II tympanoplasty, the fragements were placed parallel to long process of incus.

The annulus stapes plate in type III tympanoplasty replaces the function of the incus, crossing the promontory and reducing adhesions. The annulus stapes cartilage plate is more stable reconstruction in type III tympanoplasty than incus foreign body interpositions. The adhesions on promontory are found more often with fascia than with cartilage. The use of palisade cartilage technique bring very good functional and anatomical integrity on long-term basis. The results were equally better in butterfly and schield graft cartilage plasty.

The results of reconstructive ear surgery are affected by the type of pathology, extent of disease, condition of middle ear mucosa and the condition of Eustachain tube. In our study, cases of adhesive otitis media showed poor results. Eustachain tube function and condition of middle ear mucosa seem to affect the hearing improvement. In case of cholesteatoma and adhesive otitis media where middle ear mucosa was destroyed, we used a silastic sheet to cover the bare promontory.

Severe post-aural wound infection was seen in two cases after 3 weeks, which responded to higher antibiotics. Extrusion of cartilage was not seen in any case. Smyth since 1965 is using nasal/septal cartilage and has not encountered a single extrusion. Harris and Goodhill also did not encounter a single case of cartilage extrusion. Twelve cases of displacement of cartilage were noticed in our series. On re-exploration, this was found to be due to fibrosis around the medial end of boomrang graft which was displaced from the head of stapes. At revision surgery, this piece of cartilage was removed and conchal cartilage was used.

In type III tympanoplasty, no significant differences, based on presence or absence of superstructure of the stapes, were reported. Moreover, the use of prosthesis in comparison to the cartilage alone did not determine significant differences in the hearing threshold. Further analysis of the patient data revealed that sex and age, at the time of surgery, had no impact on postoperative hearing results. Various authors have shown that the audiologic results following cartilage tympanoplasty are comparable to those after perichondrium or fascia grafting.

The publications comparing perichondrium and cartilage, in revision type I tympanoplasty, showed, in both the groups, an ABG of less than 10 dB. Assuming that replacing a large portion of the tympanic membrane with cartilage would add stiffness and mass. Gerber compared the cartilage to fascia in a frequency-specific manner and again no significant difference was observed. Thus, postoperative hearing loss is probably due to the postoperative changes in the middle ear structures, rather than due to the material used for reconstruction. As far as cholesteatoma is concerned, our recurrence rate (3.29%) was quite low as this technique allows excellent approximation between the canal wall and reconstructed tympanic membrane to prevent retraction pocket recurrence. The indications for routine use of this more rigid material in tympanoplasty, however, remain somewhat controversial, and the impact on hearing remains to be fully elucidated.

In fact, an additional advantage of this technique might be considered the good hearing result. Overall, hearing results in our study showed a significant improvement as well as stability of the postoperative PTA-ABG. These results were related to the type of tympanoplasty. In type I showed better hearing results, the postoperative PTA-ABG (1 year after surgery) improved to 6.4 ± 2.2 dB (90% of the patients in this group had their PTA-ABG reduced to 10 dB or less). In type III tympano-plasties, no significant differences, based on presence or absence of superstructure of the stapes, were reported. Moreover, the use of prosthesis in comparison to the cartilage alone did not determine significant differences in the hearing threshold.

In our study, cartilage has been used successfully as a graft in middle ear surgery. It used to be reserved for advanced pathology because of its possible detrimental effect on post-operative hearing. The present study describes the authors' experience in 600 cases of cartilage tympanoplasty. In tympano-plasty type I, postoperative pure tone average air-bone gap was within 20 dB in 88.4% of the cases. If combined with ossiculo-plasty when the stapes were intact, 72% were within 20 dB and when the stapes were absent, 54.5% were within 20 dB. Taking rate of the graft was 95.6%. At present, the author uses cartilage graft as a first choice in tympanoplastic procedures.

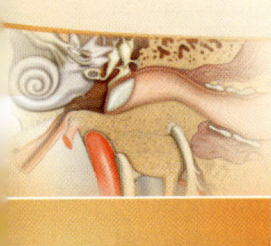

Conclusions

13

Cartilage tympanoplasty achieves good anatomical and audiologic results when pathology and status of the ossicular chain dictate the technique utilized. Significant hearing improvement was realized in each pathological group. In the atelectatic ear, cartilage allowed us to reconstruct the TM with good anatomic results compared to traditional reconstructions, which have shown high rates of retraction and failure. In cholesteatoma, cartilage tympanoplasty using the palisade technique resulted in precise reconstruction of the TM and helped reduce recurrence.

In cases of high-risk perforation, reconstruction with cartilage yielded anatomical and functional results that compared favourably to primary tympanoplasty using traditional techniques. We evaluated auditory performance following cartilage tympanoplasty for the management of tympanic membrane retraction pockets. We performed 600 patients retrospective study over a 30 years period (1980–2010) and compared preoperative and postoperative audiograms. Postoperative audiograms were better in 64% of cases, identical in 26% and worse in 10%. Cartilage tympanoplasty for the management of tympanic membrane retraction pockets has a good postoperative functional outcome. Tragal cartilage-perichondrium graft has proved very useful for reconstruction of the eardrum and ossicular defects.

The results of the present study suggest that cartilage is a good grafting material, in fact it is easily accessible, easy to fashion, resistant to negative middle ear pressures, stable (particularly in cases lacking fibrous annulus), sufficiently elastic for good sound conduction, well tolerated, resistant to resorption. Furthermore, cartilage prevents extrusion of the prosthesis, when this is used for ossicular reconstruction, and above all, it does not involve additional costs.

A potential drawback of this procedure is the graft opacity, as it may be more difficult to detect eventual residual/recurrent cholesteatoma. However, also the fascia is often not transparent.

We believe the indications for cartilage tympanoplasty (atelectatic ear, cholesteatoma, high-risk perforation) were validated by these results and hence, we strongly feel that the tragal cartilage-perichondrium graft is an ideal graft for reconstructive tympanoplasty. Hearing improvement within 15 dB of bone conduction has become almost a standard criterion for the analysis of surgical success.

It would be worthwhile, therefore, to consider cartilage-perichondrium graft as a suitable alternative to temporalis fascia. The key seems to be the use of cartilage of appropriate thickness. This would not hamper conduction of sound while protect from retraction or reperforation of the neotympanum. Perichondrium is a tough graft material showing good revascularization. The incorporation of cartilage in perichondrium as a composite would counteract negative middle ear pressure. This is of paramount importance in poor Eustachian tube function and in ears with a large perforation. We recommend the composite cartilage perichondrium graft as a perfect graft for reconstructive tympanoplasty for the following innovative reasons.

- Cartilage perichondrium appears to be ideal graft material for ears where postoperative retraction, reperforation and Eustachian tube dysfunction are of concern.
- Cartilage thickness of <0.5 mm is seen to have similar acoustic properties as the tympanic membrane.
- Cartilage–perichondrium is easy to harvest and readily available at site of surgery.
- Cartilage consists of collagen type II and is, therefore, physiologically more suitable for repair of tympanic membrane.

- Its extrusion rate is very minimum (1.19%).
- Being mesenchymal, lacks secreting glands and hair follicles, thus good for inlay grafting.
- Inexpensive, inert and non-toxic in nature.
- Immune competent and does not induce FB reaction.
- It has stiffer consistency and minimal shrinkage and lateralization.
- Natural angle of perichondrium is a perfect fit for annulus construction.

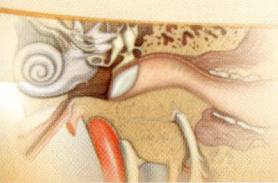

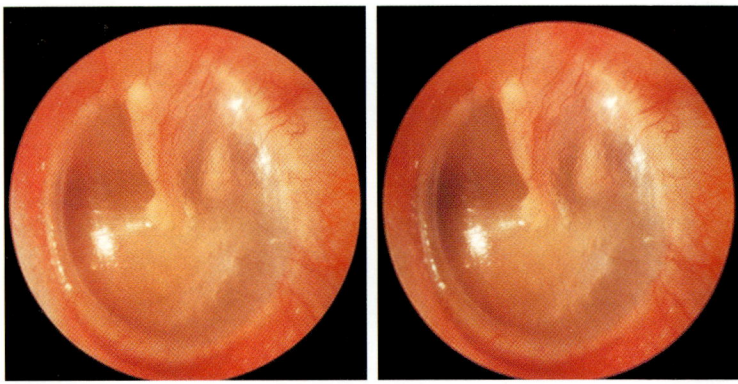

Fig. 14.1. Normal tympanic membrane

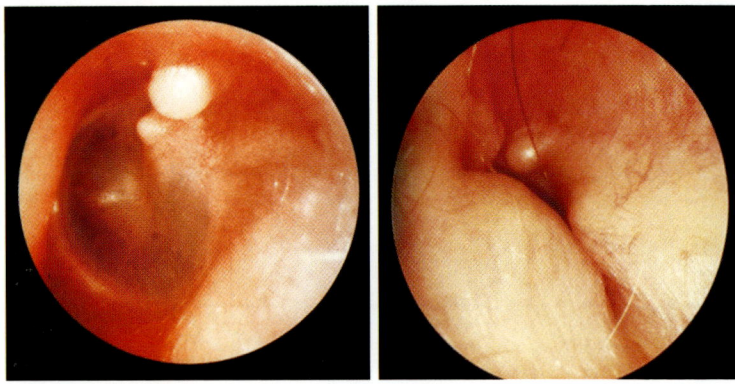

Fig. 14.2. Small exostosis   **Fig. 14.3.** Large exostoses

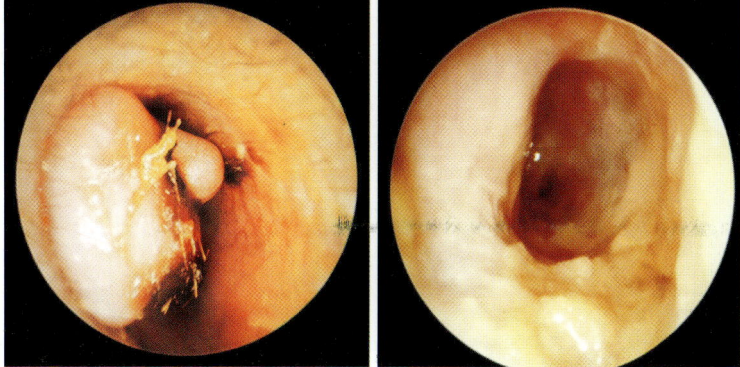

Fig. 14.4. Osteoma   **Fig. 14.5.** Otitis externa

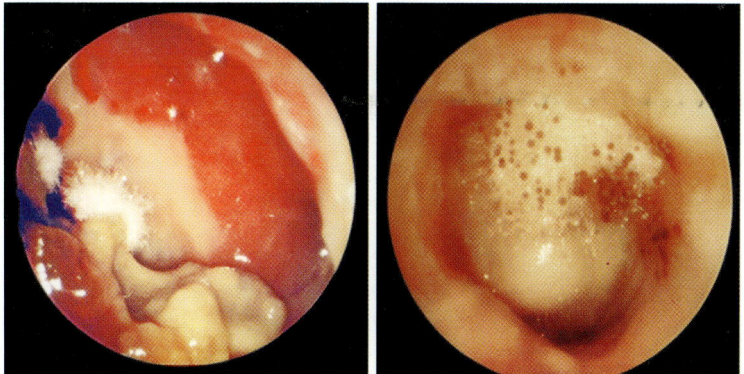

Fig. 14.6. Chronic otitis media with asso-   **Fig. 14.7.** Otomycosis with aspergillus
ciated otomycosis

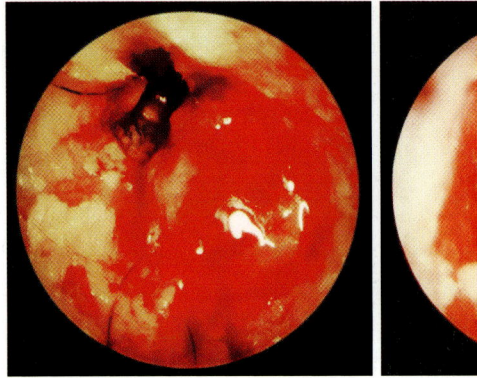

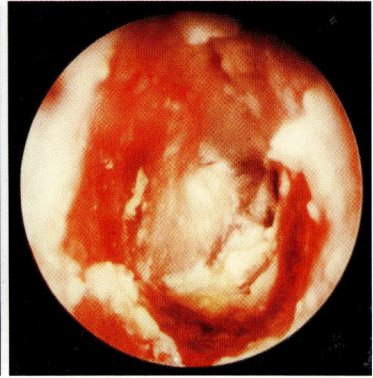

Fig. 14.8. Squamous cell carcinoma of the external auditory canal

Fig. 14.9. Otitis externa

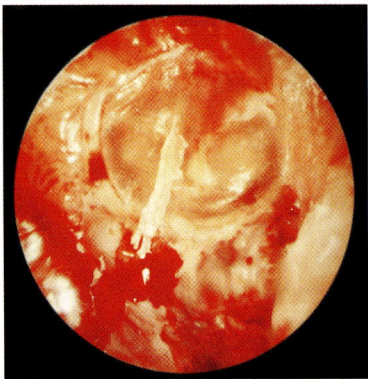

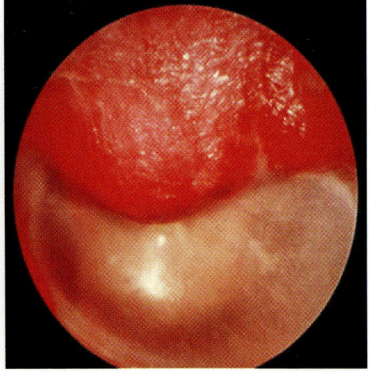

Fig. 14.10. Canal cholesteatoma following debridement

Fig. 14.11. Hemangioma of the external auditory canal

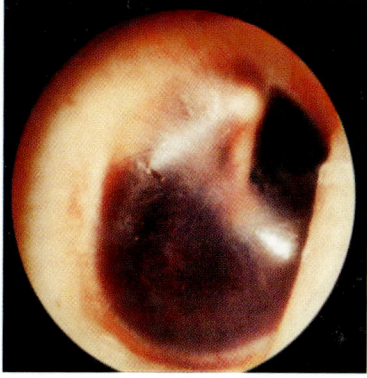

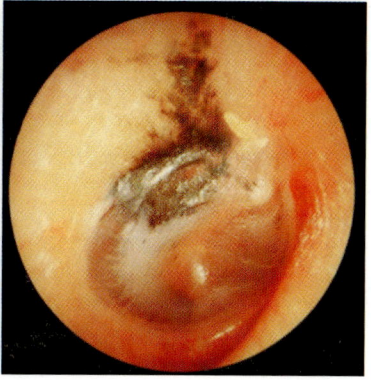

Fig. 14.12. Hemotympanum

Fig. 14.13. Lead tattoo many years following being stabbed in the ear with a pencil

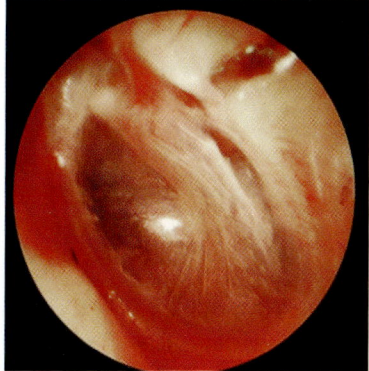

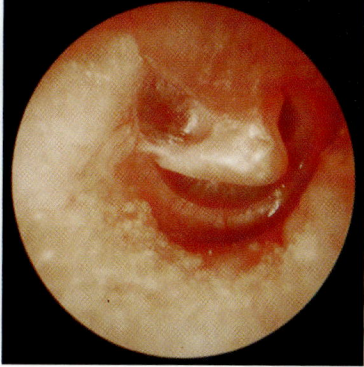

Fig. 14.14. Status post a temporal boen fracture with fracture of the scutum

Fig. 14.15. Temporal bone fracture with dislocation of the incus which is partially protruding through the tympanic membrane

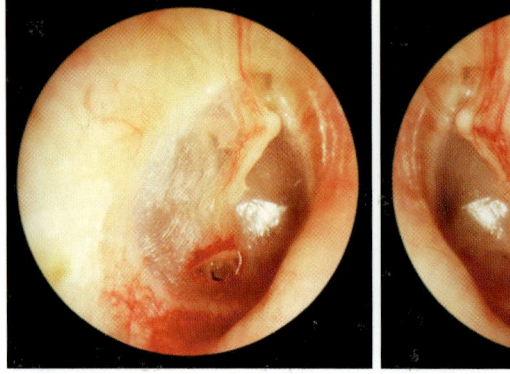

Fig. 14.16. Traumatic tympanic membrane perforation

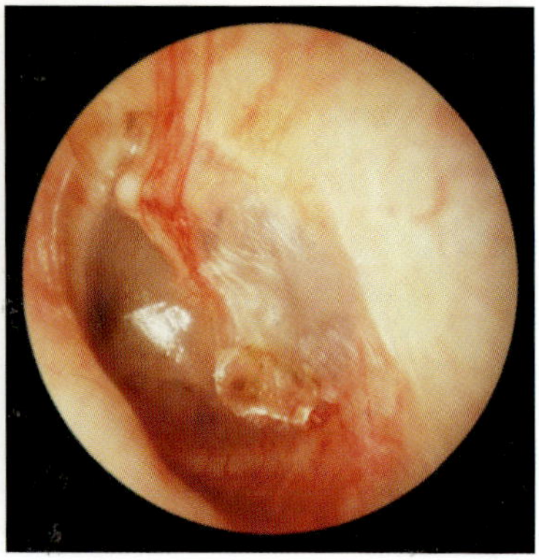

Fig. 14.17. Healing traumatic tympanic
membrane perforation

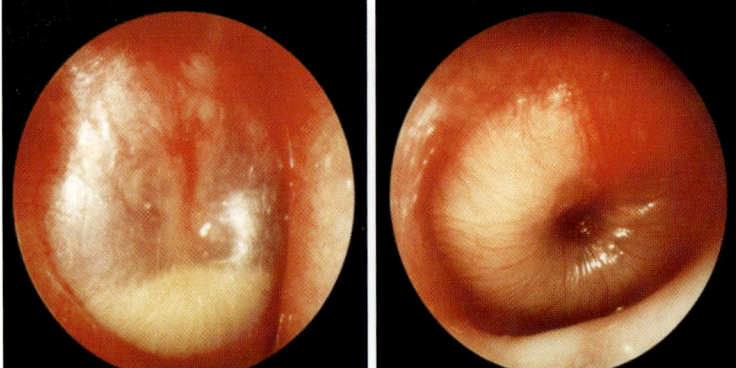

Fig. 14.18. Acute otitis media

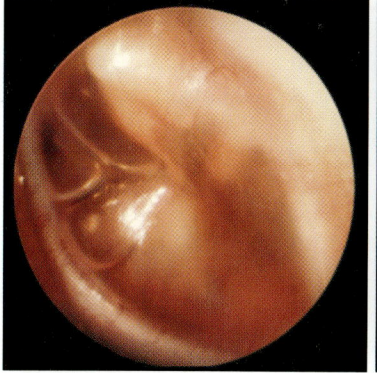

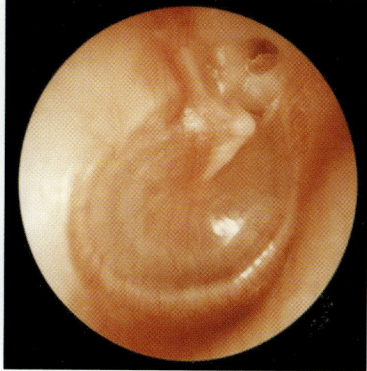

Fig. 14.19. Otitis media with effusion

Fig. 14.20. Chronic otitis media with effusion

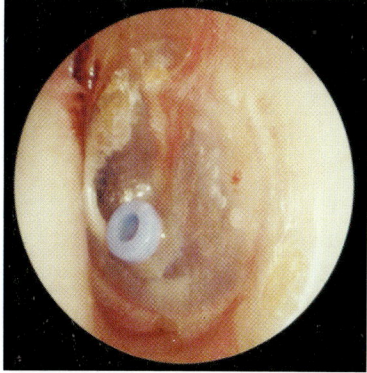

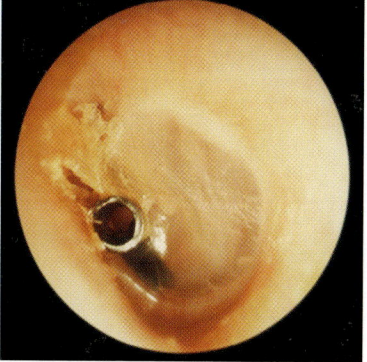

Fig. 14.21. Status post-myringotomy and PET insertion

Fig. 14.22. Status post-myringotomy and T-tube insertion

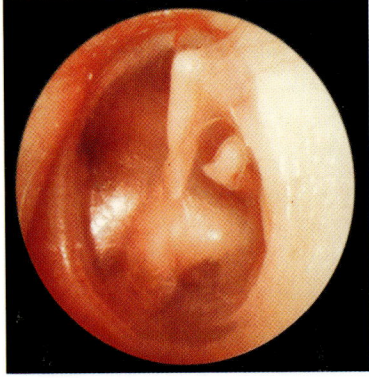

Fig. 14.23. Incudomyringopexy

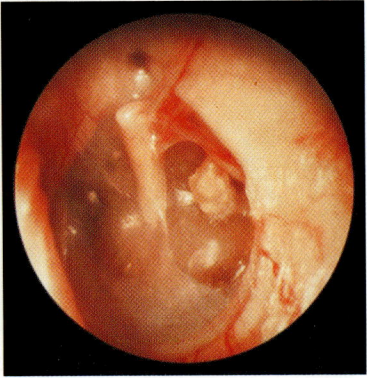

Fig. 14.24. Incudomyringopexy with early erosion of the incudostapedial joint

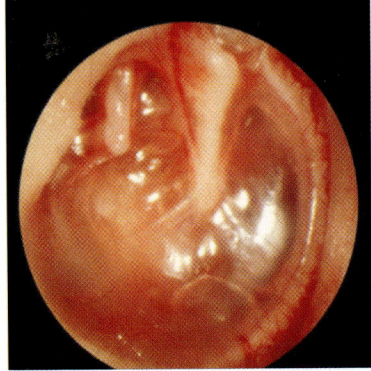

Fig. 14.25. Severe tympanic membrane atelectasis

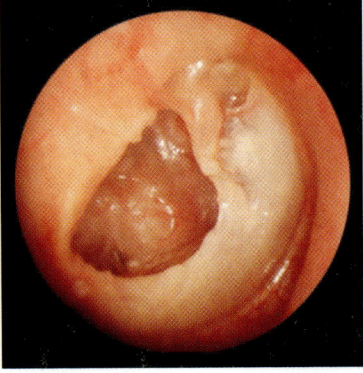

Fig. 14.26. Pars tensa retraction pocket choles-teatoma

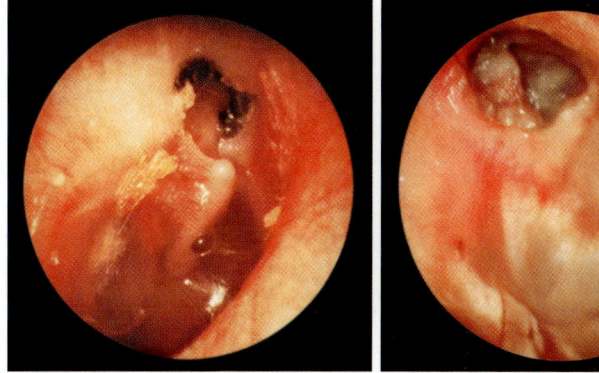

Fig. 14.27. Small attic retraction pocket choles-teatoma

Fig. 14.28. Large attic retraction pocket choles-teatoma

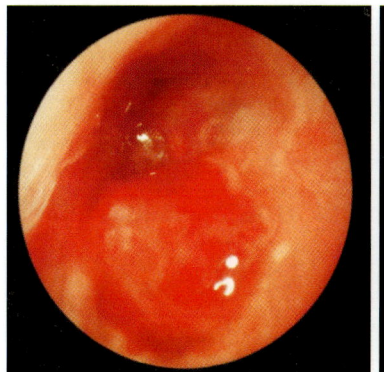

Fig. 14.29. Aural polyp

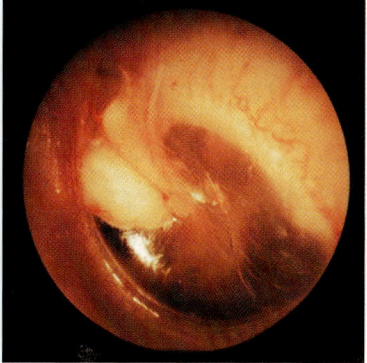

Fig. 14.30. Congenital cholesteatoma

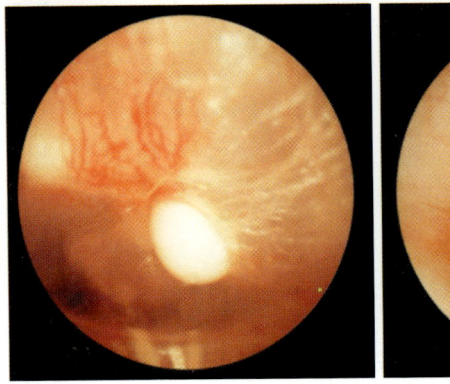

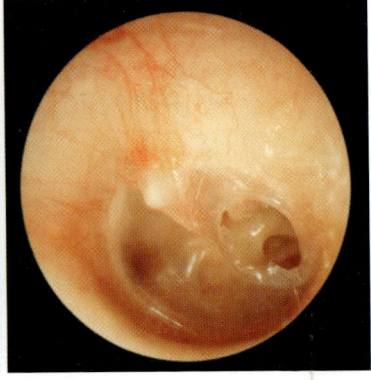

Fig. 14.31. Intratympanic cholestea-toma

Fig. 14.32. Tympanic membrane perfo-ration with exposed RW

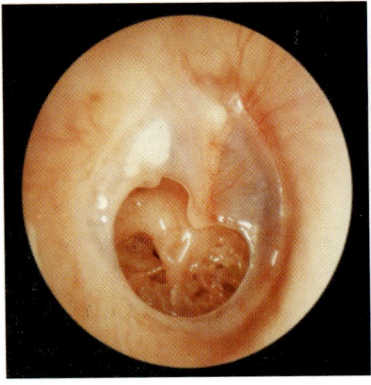

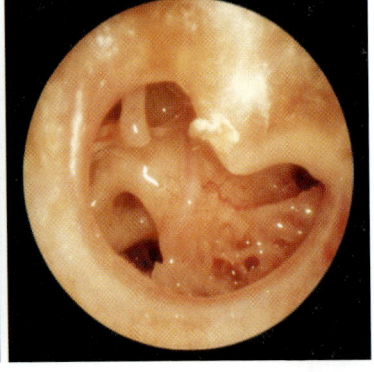

Fig. 14.33. Small central perforation

Fig. 14.34. Large subtotal tympanic membrane perforation

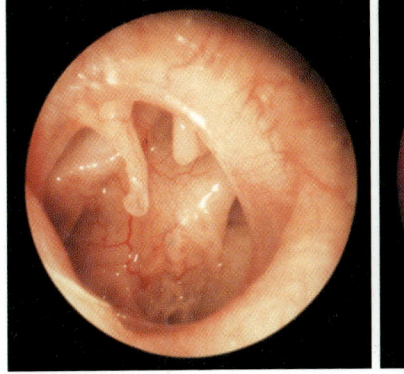 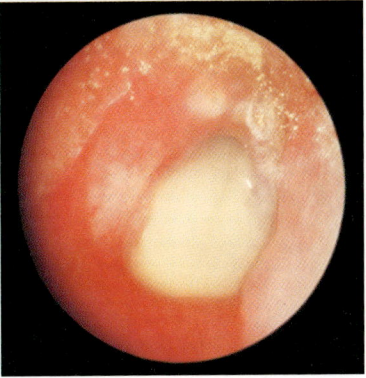

Fig. 14.35. Large total tympanic membrane perforation

Fig. 14.36. Chronic otitis media with purulent discharge

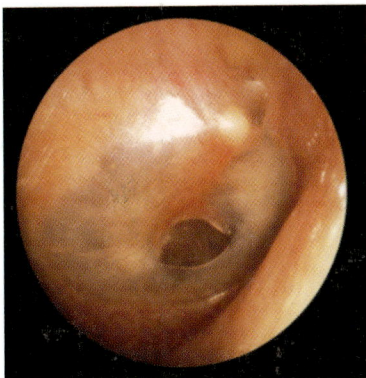 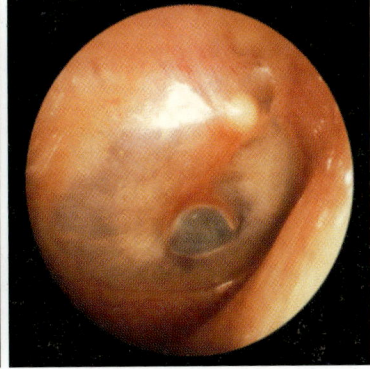

Fig. 14.37. Monomeric membrane

Fig. 14.38. Monomeric membrane with powder applied using photoshop

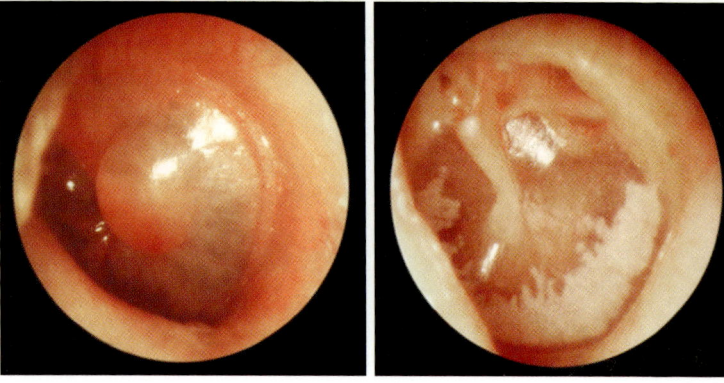

Fig. 14.39. Bullous myringitis   **Fig. 14.40.** Tympanosclerosis

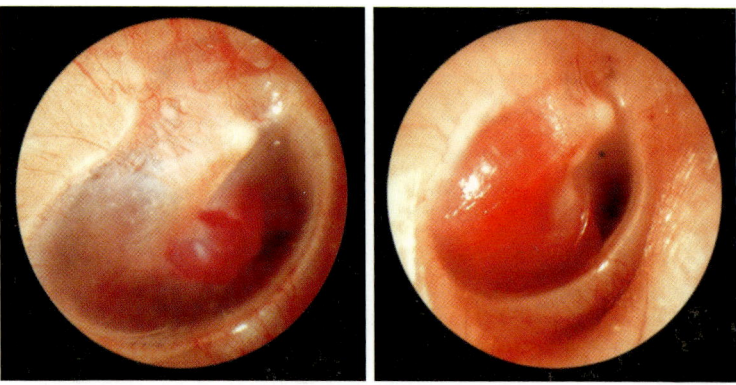

Fig. 14.41. Glomus tympanicum   **Fig. 14.42.** Glomus jugulare with middle ear extension

Bibliography

1. Abramson M. Collagenolytic activity in middle ear cholesteatoma. Annals of Otolaryngology 1989;78:112–24.
2. Altenau MN, Sheehy JL. Tympanoplasty: Cartilage prosthesis–A report of 564 cases. Laryngoscope 1978;86:895–904.
3. Andrew Don, FH Lintichum. The fate of cartilage grafts for ossicular reconstruction in tympanoplasty. Annals of Otolaryngology 1975;84: 187–91.
4. Anklesaria DM. J Laryngo 1975;77–528.
5. Austin DF. Avoiding failure in restoration of hearing with biocompatible implants. Otolaryngology Clinics of North America: 1982;15:763–71.
6. Brachman SL. Cartilage graft tympanoplasty–type III. Laryngoscope 1965;75:1452–61.
7. Diran Mikaelian. Perichondrial cartilage island graft in one stage tympano-ossiculoplasty. Laryngoscope 1986;96:237–39.
8. Elwany Somy. Histochemical study of cartilage autografts in tympanoplasty. Journal of Otolaryngology 1985;99:637–42.
9. Eviatar Abraham and Brony NY. Tragal perichondrium and cartilage in reconstructive ear surgery. Laryngoscope 1978;88(Suppl 11):1–23.
10. Gray's Anatomy. Structure of Cartilage 1985;pp.245–52.
11. Heermann J. Autografts tragal and conchal palisade cartilage and perichondrium in tympanomastoid reconstruction. Ear Nose Throat Journal 1985;71(8):344–49.
12. Hicks GW, Wright J. Use of plastipore in ossicular chain construction. Laryngoscope 1978;88:1024–33.
13. Irwin Harris, Victor Goodhill. Functional viability of tragal cartilage autografts in tympanic surgery. Laryngoscope 1967;77:1191–1203.
14. Jansen C. Cartilage tympanoplasty. Laryngoscope 1963;73:1288–1302.
15. Jansen C. Methods of ossicular reconstruction. Otolaryngology Clinics of North America 1972;5:97–109.

16. Jules Waltner. Cartilage tympanoplasty. Annals of Otolaryngology 1966;pp. 1117–23.

17. Magnham CA, East CA. Composite tragal perichondrial/cartilage autografts v/s cartilage or bone paste grafts in tympanoplasty. Clinical Otolaryngology 1991;16(6):540–42.

18. Mundada, Jaiswal. A method for ossicular reconstruction with tragal cartilage autografts. Laryngoscope 1989;99:955–62.

19. Proctor B, Proctor C, Oyal Oak. Tympanoplasty–Progress Report. Archives Otolaryngology 1970;94:94–97.

20. Pulec J, Sheehy J. Tympanoplasty: Ossicular chain reconstruction. Symposium of Tympanoplasty 1973;pp.448–64.

21. Sade J, Berco E. Bone destruction in chronic otitis media. Journal of Laryngology and Otology 1974;88:413–22.

22. Sade J, Berco E, Buyanover D, et al. Ossicular damage in chronic middle ear inflammation. Acta Otolaryngologica 1981;92:273–83.

23. Sade J, Havey A. The etiology of bone destruction in chronic otitis media. Journal of Laryngology and Otology 1974;88:139–43.

24. Schuring A, Lippy WH. Solving Ossicular problems in tympanoplasty. Laryngoscope 1983;93:1151–4.

25. Scott-Brown's Disease of Ear, Nose and Throat, 4th edn. vol. 1, Anatomy of Ear: pp. 18–19.

26. Scoot-Brown's Disease of Ear, Nose and Throat, 5th edn., vol. 3, Pathology of Inflammatory Conditions of External and Middle Ear.

27. Shea MC, Glasscock ME. Tragal cartilage as an ossicular substitute. Archives Otolaryngology 1967;86:84–91.

28. Smyth GDL. Tympanic reconstruction. Otolaryngology Clinics of North America 1972;5(1):111–25.

29. Smith BA. A glimpse of otology in Ancient world. Journal of Laryngology and Otology 1973;87:535–7.

30. Steinbach E, Pusalkar A. Long-term histological fate of cartilage in ossicular reconstruction. Journal of Laryngology and Otology 1981;95:1031–9.

31. Victor Goodhill. Tragal perichondrium and cartilage in tympanoplasty. Archives Otolaryngology 1967;85:36–47.

32. Toss M. Modification of combined approach tympanoplasty in attic cholesteatoma. Archives Otolaryngology, 1982;108:772–8.

33. John L Dornhoffer. Cartilage tympanoplasty. OCNA 2006;39: 1161–76.

34. Evitar A. Technique laryngoscope (1991). Tragal perichondrium and cartilage in reconstructive ear surgery. Laryngoscope 1978;88:1–23.

35. Gerber MJ, Mason JC, Lambet PR. Hearing results after primary cartilage tympanoplasty. Laryngoscope 2000;110:1994–5.

36. Dornhoffer JL. Hearing results with cartilage tympanoplasty. Laryngoscope 1997;107:1094–9.

37. Lubianca Neto JF. Inlay butterfly cartilage tympanoplasty (Eavey technique) modified for adult. Otolaryngol Head Neck Surg 2000;123:492–4.

38. Eavey RD. Inlay tympanoplasty: cartilage butterfly technique. Laryngoscope 1998;108:657–61.

39. Gross CW, Bassela M, Lazar RH, Long TE, Stagner S. Adipose plugue myringoplasty: an alternative to formal myringoplasty techniques in children. Otolaryngol Head Neck Surg 1989;101:617–20.

40. Levinson R. Cartilage. Perichondrial composite graft tympanoplasty in the treatment of posterior marginal and attic retractions pockets. Laryngoscope 1987;97:1069–74.

Index

Other Outstanding CBS Books in Otorhinolaryngology

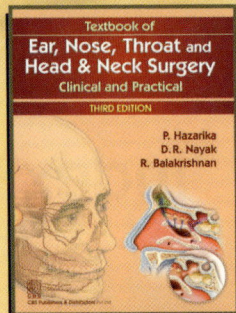
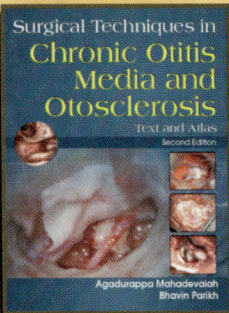
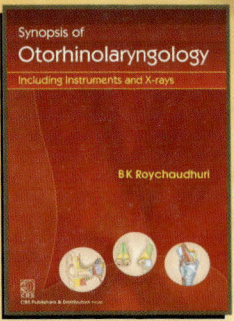

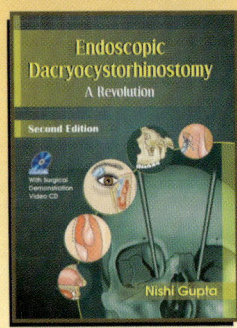
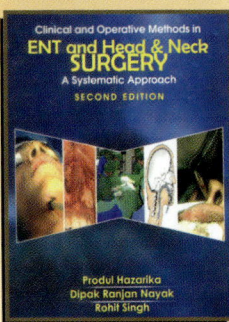
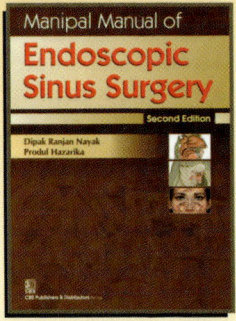

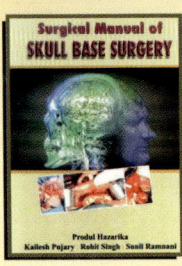
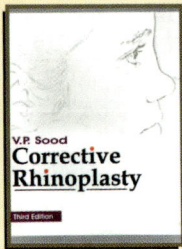
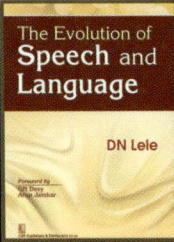
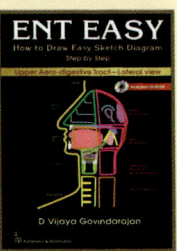

CBS Publishers & Distributors Pvt Ltd

CBS Plaza, 4819/XI Prahlad Street, 24 Ansari Road, Daryaganj, New Delhi 110 002, India. Ph: 23289259, 23266861/67, Fax: +91-11-23243014, Website: www.cbspd.com, e-mail: delhi@cbspd.com; cbspubs@airtelmail.in
Corporate Office: 204 FIE, Industrial Area, Patparganj, Delhi - 110 092, Ph: 4934 4934, Fax: 4934 4935, email: publishing@cbspd.com, publicity@cbspd.com

Branches

- Bengaluru: Seema House 2975, 17th Cross, K.R. Road, Bansaankari 2nd Stage, Bengaluru 560 070, Karnataka, Ph: 080-26771678/79, Fax: 080-26771680, e-mail: bangalore@cbspd.com
- Chennai: 7, Subbaraya Street, Shenoy Nagar, Chennai 600 030, Tamil Nadu, Ph: 044-26681266, 26680620, Fax: 044-42032115, e-mail: chennai@cbspd.com
- Kolkata: No. 6/B, Ground Floor, Rameswar Shaw Road, Kolkata - 700 014, West Bengal, Ph: 033-22891126, 22891127, 22891128, e-mail: kolkata@cbspd.com
- Kochi: 36/14 Kalluvilakam, Lissie Hospital Road, Kochi 682 018, Kerala, Ph: 0484-4059061-65, Fax: 0484-4059065, e-mail: kochi@cbspd.com
- Mumbai: 83-C, 1st floor, Dr E Moses Road, Worli, Mumbai 400 018, Maharashtra, Ph: 022-24902340/41, Fax: 022-24902342, email: mumbai@cbspd.com

Representatives

- Hyderabad: 0-9885175004 • Nagpur: 0-9021734563 • Patna: 0-9334158340 • Pune: 0-9623451994 • Vijayawada: 0-9000660880